FOOD PREFERENCES AND TASTE

THE ANTHROPOLOGY OF FOOD AND NUTRITION

General Editor: *Helen Macbeth*

FOOD PREFERENCES AND TASTE

Continuity and Change

Edited by

Helen Macbeth

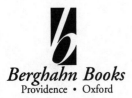

Berghahn Books
Providence • Oxford

First published in 1997 by

Berghahn Books

© 1997 Helen Macbeth

Library of Congress Cataloging-in-Publication Data

```
Food preference and taste : continuity and change / edited by Helen
Macbeth.
      p.   cm. -- (The anthropology of food and nutrition ; v. 2)
   Includes bibliographical references (p.        ) and index.
   ISBN 1-57181-958-4 (hardcover : alk. paper). -- ISBN 1-57181-970-3
(pbk. : alk. paper)
   1. Food. 2. Food preferences. 3. Food consumption. 4. Taste.
5. Nutritional anthropology.   I. Macbeth, Helen M.  II. Series.
GN407.F68  1997
306.4--dc21                                              97-28668
                                                             CIP
```

British Library Cataloguing in Publication Data

A catalogue record for this book is available from the British Library.

Printed in the United States on acid-free paper.

CONTENTS

FIGURES AND MAPS

Figures

Maps

TABLES

FOREWORD

Mary Douglas

It is an honour to be invited to say a few words about the International Commission on the Anthropology of Food (I.C.A.F.) at the beginning of this volume, and also a great kindness on the part of Helen Macbeth to give me a little sense of involvement in the flourishing work of I.C.A.F. (Europe) which Igor de Garine and his international colleagues have done so much to build up.

It must have been in 1977, soon after I had arrived in New York, that I received a letter from Ravindra Khare suggesting that he and I should found a new committee within the framework of the International Union of Anthropological and Ethnological Sciences (I.U.A.E.S.). It was fair in a way that he should have thought of asking me, because I was just starting a programme on the social aspects of food for the Russell Sage Foundation. We did not know each other and he did not know that he could hardly have chosen a colleague with less administrative or entrepreneurial flair. I have much pride and pleasure in looking back on a partnership I never would have predicted. If we did put anything together, it was thanks to his consistent vision and resolute determination, both always belied by his modest demeanour and sense of humour.

The first thing we did was to organise in 1978 a panel on the anthropology of food and food problems at the Tenth International Congress of the I.U.A.E.S. in Delhi. I edited the volume *Constructive Drinking* (1987) on the basis of those meetings. We also had a conference in the fabulous Burg Wartenstein organised for us by the Wenner Gren Foundation. We went to Rome to get support from the Food and Agriculture Organisation. We had informal meetings in New York and with another panel at the I.U.A.E.S. Congress in Vancouver. We could have done nothing without the support of Lita Osmundsen, the Director of the Wenner Gren Foundation in New York, and of Clemens Heller, Director of the Maison des Sciences de l'Homme in Paris. We had some wonderful colleagues, including Gretel Pelto, Lenore Manderson, Dwight Heath, Gerald Mars, and Igor de Garine who founded the European branch. We discussed wonderfully interesting topics such as the four humours used in medicine, food used in strategies of rejection, social pressures on women's diet.

At that time the topic of famine and nutrition was being studied very seriously, with good reason, but the social aspects of food were neglected. There was, and perhaps still is, a tendency to think that the only things that can be said about the social aspects of food have to be funny or frivolous. The reason may be that it is extremely difficult to combine the cultural with the biological approach. Thanks to Igor de Garine, his strong development of the European branch and his fruitful collaboration with Geoffrey Harrison, a real dialogue has grown up between biological and other anthropologists.

I was actually present at the Oxford conference on which this book is based and was happy to observe what lively and highly specialised sets of scholars have been working together on the anthropology of food all these years. Their originality and ability to spark off important issues has developed a whole new field, as is evident from the essays here.

PREFACE

The International Commission on the Anthropology of Food (I.C.A.F.) is a commission launched under the auspices of the International Union of Anthropological and Ethnological Sciences (I.U.A.E.S.). This volume arises out of the fourth international symposium of the European section of I.C.A.F., which was held in July 1993 at the Pauling Human Sciences Centre, Oxford University.

The topic is of interest not only to biological and social anthropologists but also to psychologists, zoologists and physiologists, as well as to all concerned with food production and retailing. In this volume contributions from specialists in quite different academic disciplines have been deliberately brought together rather than scattered in the literature of disparate specialisms.

I.C.A.F. is grateful for the support and encouragement of Berghahn Books, who also published the proceedings of their second European symposium. The Editor thanks the contributors to the symposium and to the volume, as well as Ros Odling Smee of the Pauling Centre, and Sue Lawry, Aleks Collingwood, Eleanor McDonald, Shelley Baldwin and Alex Green, all graduates of Oxford Brookes University, who contributed in many ways to the organisation of the symposium, administration of contributions requested and received, and editorial assistance on the word-processed texts. The Economic and Social Research Council grant (number I 439 26 9307) for the conference is acknowledged.

H.M.M., 1997

1. FOOD PREFERENCES AND TASTE
AN INTRODUCTION

Helen Macbeth and *Sue Lawry*

Setting the Scene

It is evident from the span of literature on the subject that the topic of food preferences and taste has many perspectives. However, the information has been scattered in the journals and books of different academic disciplines, simplified in the public media or creatively represented by those involved in or with the food industries. This book attempts to address some of the complexity of processes involved in human food choices. While cross-disciplinary cooperation is desirable, truly *inter*disciplinary biosocial research is rare, if not non-existent, because the ultimate objectives of any individual study are likely to be perceived either in biological or in socioeconomic terms. Human food is an excellent topic for multidisciplinary discourse. It generally avoids the mutual misunderstandings of some oversimplified polemics, while it fosters real interest in the interaction of such subjects as dietary values, high and low status foods, biochemistry, religious avoidances, hunger, commensality and nutritional health, in researchers studying any one of these angles. At the same time, human interest in food is such that the 'general public' seem to have an insatiable appetite for books and articles on food, either to read or to give at Christmas. Furthermore, as authors in cross-disciplinary collections should avoid the jargon peculiar to their discipline, their papers, unlike much academic writing, are likely to be accessible to a wider audience.

This volume does not aspire to unravel all the component parts, but through a series of chapters written by specialists from different disciplines, the objective is to allow different perspectives to be published together, so that readers from whatever background can gain information from a diversity of viewpoints.

There is, however, one particular difficulty in discussing this topic in the English language – that is the ambiguity in the word 'taste'. Leaving aside its non-food extension to personal ideas on the aesthetics of anything and its use as a synonym for sophistication, there is still ambiguity. There are the biochemical reactions and the attitudes to those reactions; even the physiological processes of the sensory perceptions are divided between gustation and olfaction. Gustation concerns sensations from the tongue, which, as is widely understood, can distinguish between sweet, sour, salty and bitter. Less popularly known is the sensation called *umami*, as the tongue reacts to protein stimulation. However, with increasing research into these reactions, it has been found that there are many substances that cannot be easily classified within these categories. What is more, as Hladk and Simmen (1996) suggest, sensory integration might be best described as a continuum of sensations rather than by discrete categories of taste. So, the question has been reopened and remains unresolved. Olfaction is due to sensory reactions in the nasopharyngeal region, and although linked to one nerve, the range of diversity perceived seems to be infinite. This may be called 'flavour', a useful word to distinguish olfaction from 'taste' as limited to gustatory sensations. There is, furthermore, the trigeminal system, which is the reaction to chemical stimuli, such as the 'heat' sensation of pepper or the 'cooling' sensation of peppermint.

Whilst use of the words 'food preferences' can overcome this language problem, there are differences of emphasis in the following chapters such that both preferences and taste are included in the title of this book.

What is more, it is hoped that the phrase 'food preferences and taste' indicates the need for the crossdisciplinary approach. Indeed, discussion of the aetiology of food preferences has not escaped the arguments nicknamed the 'Nature/Nurture debate'. Macbeth (1989) has suggested that decades of academic controversy have been wasted on the perception of 'Nature' and 'Nurture' as two sides of some dichotomy. Research on the activity of biochemical substances affecting, and affected by, mind and emotions has developed the comprehension of complex multifactorial neurological interactions. Furthermore, the increased knowledge of how DNA only codes for the order of available amino acids in protein formation has shown that even biochemistry is due to a fundamental interaction of genetic and non-genetic factors. In humans, this complexity is further embellished by the capacity of the human brain not only for actions and emotions, but also for language and concepts. Such features are acquired through socialisation, and the flexibility of the human mind has led to infinite variations of cultures within which such socialisation takes place. Rather slowly in the wake of such understanding of multiple interactions, biosocial cooperation is now receiving academic respectability, even though individual specialists steeped in the different 'cultures' of their disciplines tend to pursue answers to quite different questions, involving quite different methodologies. In such a situation one cannot expect integration of academic pursuits (Chapman, 1990). Yet, collation, without antagonism, of perspectives by sociological and biological scientists allows a richer comprehension of the component factors within this complexity.

Even children in a family or school are aware of individual differences in food preferences, but adults realise that their own attitudes to some foods have changed considerably since childhood. Such changes with age coexist with the early development of some likes and dislikes that persist throughout adulthood. Research into the origin of gustatory perceptions has concluded that newborn infants perceive sweet, sour and bitter immediately, but perhaps develop perception of salt a few months after birth. Reactions suggesting distaste on receiving sour or bitter ingredients are regularly recorded in research on neonates, while sweet tastes seem to give pleasure. This has led to the debates of whether or not these perceptions are genetic in origin, which miss the point of the essential interaction of the genetic and non-genetic. What is clear is that gustatory sensations develop very early. On the other hand, olfactory likes and dislikes seem to develop through experiences and associations throughout life.

That there are culinary differences between different cultures and regions is now popularly proclaimed and to some extent anchored by the publication of regional cookbooks, while the more ethnographic writing on food has tended to concentrate on the social aspects of the meals, the commensality, gender roles, cooking practices, and the symbolism of particular foodstuffs. Nevertheless, it has long been recognised that there is great variation in individual food preferences, both between and within populations. Pilgrim, in the early 1960s, distinguished patterns in relation to within-population characteristics, not only of age, but also of education, or 'sophistication', regional and cultural differences, etc. From a decade of studies on men in the U.S. armed forces, he perceived little secular change with time, despite 'advertising and changed marketing techniques' (Pilgrim, 1961: 442). Such temporal stability does not appear to be supported by several authors in this book (González, Valagao, McDonaugh) who describe studies where social changes correlate with changes in food choices. A typical cause of change arises from the popularisation of scientific knowledge about nutrition and its health consequences. As science is a dynamic process, the specialist conclusions change, followed only later by the popularisation of those conclusions.

Where the economic situation allows, fashion also affects preferences, for example in the search for the exotic or the homemade as discussed by James (in press). The fashion mechanism is implicated in Campbell's (1987) discussion of consumerism. However, such changes with fashions are only available to those whose socioeconomic and ecological situations allow such choices. González (this volume) reports that the labouring classes in western Andalucia, who until recently had few choices, state preferences for exactly what they do eat, while a consumerism, which she discusses, is found particularly in the middle classes and the *nouveaux riches*. De Garine (this volume) makes a similar point that for some traditional African societies, where periods of hunger are not infrequent, security, not boredom, is found in the regular consumption of the cereal staple. From the limited range of foods of poverty, through food scarcity to the extreme situation of famine, there appears to be a scale of changes as generally avoided wild foods are sought and consumed. Below, Huss-Ashmore and Johnston show how selections of wild alternatives depend on folk knowledge of nutrition, but then, as conditions worsen, any bulk items are consumed which ease the pain of hunger.

From such comments arises the idea of an economic U-shaped curve, in regard to change and continuity: those economically able to do so seek novelty and new taste stimulation, while those with less access to choice are glad just to have enough of the familiar basic foods. When even these fail there is change again, but through necessity not preference. This necessity may not only derive from unfavourable ecological circumstances, but also from wars, sociopolitical inequalities, etc., that interrupt the continuity of production and consumption; the disruption in food habits caused by migration should also be described as necessity when traditional ingredients are not available in the new situation. Changes due to such *necessities* may in due course become encoded into the *preferences* of the people concerned or their offspring.

It is evident, then, that ethnographic, economic and ecological settings must always be included in discussions of change and continuity in human food preferences and taste. Disjunctures in life situation are very likely to cause change, but diversity is also sought when life conditions are affluent and secure. At the same time, biochemistry underlies these processes, not *determining* the outcome, but affecting the flexibility of the responses. Such biochemistry, which, as with all biology, is subject to evolutionary processes and within-life changes, must also be considered neither immutable nor homogeneous throughout all humanity.

Framework of the Chapters

In the following chapters several authors point out that the topic as a whole lacks systematic research and academic integration. It is almost certainly over-ambitious to expect that the latter can ever be attained. Nevertheless in this volume persistent themes cut across most chapters. It has been hard to identify an ideal order of chapters and the editor has chosen a framework that starts with research on non-human primates to indicate one route to understanding evolutionary origins of human taste perception and its use as a successful survival strategy.

Hladik, indicating the complexity, shows that the process is not merely a correspondence between taste qualities (salt, bitter, sour and sweet) and taste-bud responses, but also the recognition of a medley of sensory characteristics to provide the taste 'signature' of each substance. Using non-human primates and human populations as examples he suggests that adaptive strategies exist in the negative responses to salty and bitter tastes, but considers that the benefits of sensitivity to sour and sweet may be because of positive preferences. After putting his discussion into human context by comparing sensitivity to salt in two contrasted populations, the Inuit of Greenland and the pygmies from Zaire, he reviews research on taste sensitivity in non-human primate species. He admits to problems of interpretation in using behavioural studies of non-human primates for studying human sensitivity, but believes that choice is made at a level above the threshold of taste (supra-threshold), and so reveals the hedonic dimension. Emphasising the value of a volume of this cross-disciplinary nature, Hladik stresses the need for more research into the complex biological and sociocultural relationships involved in the expression of taste responses and food preferences.

In Chapter 3 Simmen describes a study of neotropical primates and their ability to discriminate between levels of soluble sugar. Phylogenetic constraints rather than adaptive responses are considered in the context of whether a taste recognition threshold automatically governs expression of preference in relation to dietary niche. Species of similar body weight have similar basal energy needs, and therefore, Simmen argues, diversity in diets may reflect not only different adaptive strategies in relation to niche, but also the expression of preferences. A relationship between feeding strategy and taste discrimination is postulated, since those species which can distinguish sugars at the lowest level travel furthest to secure them and consume the greatest diversity of fruits with high sugar content. What is the role of the hedonic value of taste in feeding behaviour and what is the relative importance of sensory reward compared to satisfaction of energy needs? Reflections on a similar issue are found later in the volume in the context of culturally determined expressions of preference either for satiety gained from familiar foods, or for novel taste stimuli where these can be afforded.

Rolls, in the next chapter, provides detailed information regarding the neuronal responses which affect the selection of quantity and variety of foods due to visual and taste stimuli. He shows that if an individual is satiated with a particular food, the neuronal response is switched off, and this food will be refused. Yet, a new food may well be selected, preceded by the appropriate neuronal signals. As 'pleasantness' decreases with satiety, neurons are part of the food reward system and thus contribute to regulation of intake. He points to the interesting paradox that an evolutionary advantage which ensured consumption of the full range of nutrients, when available, may today be disadvantageous, leading to overeating and obesity. At the other extreme, which he illustrates with an example in a refugee camp, that boredom with a much repeated food item may lead to its rejection and the selection of a less nutritious alternative.

However satiety is not the only mechanism for rejection, and Schiefenhövel writes on the facial expression and physiological mechanisms triggered by disgust. Not only is the physiology described with a clarity accessible to non-biologists, but he elegantly relates this understanding to the acquisition of disgust emotions through cultural stimuli. He exemplifies how this kind of revulsion is frequently used about what other ethnic groups eat and drink, and that through such aversions ethnic groups effectively attain different ecological niches. He supports his case with brief ethnographic data from different Melanesian islands. This makes an interesting comparison to Simmen's discussion of the exploitation of different environmental niches by different primate species. In one brief chapter, detailed biological information is linked with ethnographic data from his research area to suggest a concept of great ecological significance.

Rozin et al., in Chapter 6, also consider processes of adaptive success, rooted in mammalian biology, as preadaptations for cultural processes. They too concentrate on the disgust emotion, which once protected the body from poisonous substances but has been elaborated, they argue, into a socially constructed behaviour which protects the 'soul' from pollution and aids assimilation of cultural rules. The ontogenesis of disgust is charted from core disgust which essentially relates to offensive substances, through animal origin disgust, which reminds us of aspects of our animal natures, and interpersonal disgust which is related to undesirable objects associated with other people. This last may serve as an ethnic or outgroup marker. They finally refer to moral disgust, rooted in anger, contempt and fear of moral taint. A question left unanswered is whether disgust is, then, the emotion of civilisation, culture's most powerful prohibition that internalises the rejection of offensive thoughts and values, as well as of materials. This provocative chapter should stimulate debate.

While the physiological processes in this complex biosocial relationship are undeniable, cultural effects on food preferences, operating through socialisation and experience, are so diverse that the possibilities for ethnographic information are limitless. The topic returns to preference rather than disgust in the chapter by Huss-Ashmore and Johnston, who after a useful survey of relevant literature pursue the theme of selection in the context of severe conditions of scarcity. As coping strategies have to be part of the overall adaptive repertoire of pre-industrial populations, the authors probe the biological, psychological and cultural factors which govern the selection of wild plants as famine foods, to ascertain whether choices appear to be made on the basis of taste or because of social and ecological factors. Choices are shown to progress, as famine worsens, from taste preferences through notions of nutritive value to feelings of fullness. In the worst conditions, this last may well override bad taste, known toxicity, cultural proscription and even feelings of disgust. If disgust, as Rozin et al. had suggested, is the emotion of civilisation, it is implicit that 'civilisation' can be overridden by the reaction to severe environmental stress and distress. Prior to acute famine, the perception of shortage is probably a reaction to the lack of preferred foods rather than a complete absence of food. So, preferences are expressed as an equation, which balances the benefits of nutritional value, taste and satiety against the costs of time spent, energy expended and probable toxicity. Ethnographic studies in Africa and North America are cited to confirm that these are indeed strategies.

That food scarcity can lead to the adoption of an alternative also features in the following chapter by Messer, which is concerned with one food item, the potato. The historical, ecological and socioeconomic influences on the geographic spread of the potato provide the context for her arguments on the development of food preferences in different populations. Her arguments develop Mintz's (1996) essay on change in food habits and the relevance of external pressures in the mutability of taste cultures. The potato is an interesting example as it only reached Europe in the sixteenth century and was at first viewed with repulsion, but its agricultural advantages in a diversity of climates fostered its spread in times of scarcity and war, and in many European regions it became a staple. This had opposing effects on preferences: for the poor that depended on it, it became encoded in their culture, but for others it either became associated with poverty and despised or was integrated into local cuisines and acclaimed. In modern times pride in the potato is claimed by several ethnicities. In Messer's discussion of European potato dishes different national preferences are displayed in the cuisine, but the potato is the common ingredient. Her discussion encompasses examples around the world and does not neglect to mention potato processing for fast foods.

Cultural diversity has already been referred to and ethnographies form the evidence for such diversity. Ethnographies are the data on which much of social anthropology is based but their relevance to biological anthropology is not infrequent. The next six chapters relate specific case studies, three of which are within Europe, one in Nepal, one in Thailand, and one concerns Iranian migrants to Britain. The population samples on which González writes live in western Andalucia, and were originally chosen because of certain environmental features. As it turned out there was little to report on differences due to ecology, and consideration was then given to differences by age, gender and socioeconomic position in regard to food preferences and intake, all of which were shown to be significant. In an area where some new food habits have been acquired due to new retailing outlets, and where other food habits are traditional rural Andalucian, including consumption of some wild foods, data were obtained on the composition of the diet, processing methods, the origins of food, the attitudes to food, and the foods used for special occasions. Although there were no major differences in intake by locality, preference was almost always expressed for the foods provided by the local environment, fish by the sea and pork products near the pig farms.

A significant finding is that while the labouring classes express preference for what they do eat, and satiety and abundance are their dietary aspirations, the middle classes and the *nouveaux riches* seek the prestige foods which are still symbols of élitisim even now that they are available to all. A consumerism that persistently acquires new objects of desire is associated with these classes much more than with either the poor or the truly élite aristocracy. Only a few gender differences could be identified, but considerable attention is given to age differences.

Valagao's study of the changes in eating habits in the Alto Douro, the Port wine producing area of northern Portugal, also shows that preferences can only be expressed where economic and social change bring the luxury of choice. Before the 1960s the monoculture of the vine had polarised society into a powerful landowning élite with a rich variety of food choices and the mass of poor labourers with a monotonous diet. The author describes the factors of war in the colonies, migration, revolution at home and the increasing prominence of industrial and service sectors of the economy, which inevitably led to the rejection of the previous rural poverty and oppressive employment practices in the vineyards. At the same time, the availability of a wider variety of mass produced goods, the increase in modern kitchen equipment and the easing of the stranglehold of vineyard working patterns allowed an increasing diversity of meal times, food types and patterns of commensality. However, in the midst of change, one aspect of continuity or tradition remained in the *merenda*, or mid-afternoon snack. Previously a break in the labouring day governed by imposed work patterns, it has now become a transition meal between work or school and leisure activities; it consists of highly prized items which express the luxury of 'time off'. *Merenda* is a symbol of freedom to choose in a society where food traditions and modernity coexist.

At the time of the conference from which this volume arises, there were much reported discussions about sovereignty, federalism, and the European Union meetings at Maastricht. The debates were well featured in the media, reflecting the intense feelings many people have about nationality and ethnicity. The processes of socialisation that give rise to such feelings are not discussed in this volume, but the use of food preference to demarcate ethnic groups has been referred to. The following chapter by Macbeth and Green considers whether, in two neighbouring populations either side of the Franco-Spanish border, expressions of food preferences by teenagers indicate that cultural markers of national identity and division are stronger than a supposed European, or even international, teenage culture. Unlike previous research which contrasts the young persons' subculture as a whole with that of the adult population (e.g., James, 1979; González, this volume), this research into food choices shows significant differences between French and Spanish teenagers in both food preferences and concepts of the health properties of food items. The teenagers in question live in the Cerdanya valley in the eastern Pyrenees where residents may in different contexts consider themselves to be French, Spanish, Catalan or Cerdan, or certain combinations of these, revealing the complexity of disentangling the multilayered nature of identity.

Food selection and consumption may be based on many factors unrelated to taste, such as availability, cost, hygiene or snobbery. Meanwhile the development of preferences is shown in this volume to have a complex aetiology, one aspect of which is clearly enculturation reflecting home experiences as well as national and ethnic identity. A development of González's point about the use of food preferences as expressions of identity is the suggestion that as the European borders become more open, differences in food habits may increasingly be used to symbolise differences in nationality to strengthen the notional border. The question is, perhaps, whether the powerful international retailing businesses will affect, or will find ways to reflect, traditional food choices. This thread is picked up in the final chapter of the volume in terms of pride in local traditions in the presence of modern influences.

An element not discussed so far is that most cultures have traditional beliefs concerning the health values of certain foods which also affect attitudes to different foods. Concepts about the health values of foods are socially interesting and some have long histories, but increasingly in Europe one feels that such concepts are for some people becoming an important, quasi-scientific belief system unattached to other religious beliefs. It is interesting, therefore, to turn to a region where explicit food prohibitions are traditionally linked to religious and social systems. McDonaugh examines the changes in the prohibition on eating buffalo meat over a thirteen-year period amongst the Tharu of the Dang valley in south-west Nepal, in the context of hierarchy and purity. In this society, rules concerning food and commensality are some of the most important markers of status and purity that define the boundaries of castes in South Asian society.

It is therefore all the more remarkable that the consumption of one meat, previously associated only with lower-ranking castes, is increasing in a middle-ranking group like the Tharu. The author outlines a changing situation where there has been a general relaxation of traditional caste food practices. Among the Tharu, status does not rest entirely upon notions of relative purity, and with changes in road access and politics a new outward-looking attitude has promoted the increased selection of buffalo meat. He reports on a situation of change where a new, radical, egalitarian element exists in slightly uneasy juxtaposition with the continuity of caste hierarchy. The fact that buffalo is euphemistically known as 'big goat' points to the human ability to loosen the bonds of social acceptability by a judicious use of reclassification.

Moving further east to a population of small scattered hill communities in Thailand, Hubert, in her study of the Yao, shows that classification of food items, meal types and associated behaviours are constrained by this society's notions of space in both the temporal world and the world of the ancestors. Men express a preference for strong 'virile' foods such as meat, blood and alcohol, and women express a preference for foods considered ladylike such as fruit and noodles, i.e., bland, tender, stewed or boiled foods. They cannot do otherwise but express these preferences because they represent their respective positions: men as the 'bridge' between the visible world of the household and the invisible world of the ancestors, and women as the civilised heart of the household where food is cooked using proper utensils and proper table manners are employed. Children occupy an intermediate position, also held by the swiddens (forest gardens) which mediate between nature which gives and humans who consume. Children may consume either raw or grilled foods outside, but by adolescence they must take on the food preferences of their sex. Within the home raw food may only be consumed at a sacrifice symbolising the incorporation of the ancestors into the civilised heart of the household. The purpose of food, and so preferences, for the Yao, therefore, is to balance and nourish relations between the temporal world and the nether world, to ensure the health and prosperity which can only be secured by 'feeding' the ancestors appropriate foods. Hubert's fieldwork was carried out in 1969/70, and it would be interesting to know how the forces of change, access and politics, significant in the previous chapter, have affected food choices in this society.

People experience change not only when it occurs within their own society, but when they migrate from their native land to a new country with a totally different culture. In regard to food preferences and taste Harbottle interviewed migrants from Iran to Britain – a change not only of society but also of ecology which affects the availability (or cost) of many food items. It is a common feature of migration that 'ethnic' cuisine is retained as far as possible after migration, but some ingredients may have to be changed. The views of individual Iranian migrants on the development of their own food preferences are integrated by Harbottle into a useful discussion of the complementary perspectives on taste provided by both social and biological scientists and the importance of the cross-disciplinary approach.

Appropriately, the last word goes to de Garine, the Commissioner of the International Commission on the Anthropology of Food. He also stresses the complexity of the subject of taste, and points out that, notwithstanding our biological inheritance, food preferences and aversions are acquired within a cultural framework. In studying rain forest and savanna populations in Cameroon, all small-scale traditional societies, he addresses the criteria which govern food selection and the expression of preferences and aversions. The two forest populations with a more than adequate, healthy diet harvest fish from the sea and game from the forest, but consider the gathering of wild plants a sign of poverty and hunger in a situation where preferences are often expressed in terms of skill in preparation and health values. In contrast the two savanna populations have a monotonous, less secure diet and regular shortage is experienced. Here descriptions of 'good taste' mean the same thing as 'most filling' – a point similar to that made by Huss-Ashmore and Johnston. By valuing satiety, a monotonous diet is accepted. In these societies the common staple, or 'cultural superfood' is most often consumed, is recognised as most commonly consumed, has a positive image and is preferred. This is reminiscent of González's point that the poor express preference for exactly what they do eat. The forest populations have been exposed to Western influences for the longest time and feel most secure about their traditional food practices as proud cultural markers, whereas the savannah populations have less confidence and tend to relate traditional practices to failure and backwardness. De Garine concludes that familiarity and satiety are valued in traditional societies, whereas the idea that monotony leads to boredom and rejection may only be valid in prosperous, industrialised societies, where individuals require novelty (a point also made by González). However, the examples provided by Rolls and Schiefenhövel in this volume demonstrate other perspectives on this. There may be a difference, Rolls suggests, between the repetition of strong flavoured foods and the repetition of staples which are mostly bland. De Garine reminds us that if we are to avoid making hasty generalisations about food preferences based only on modern, urban, industrialised societies we must continue to study non-Western food systems.

Overview and Challenge

Among these chapters on taste, preference and disgust, interesting themes recur; for example, socialisation, identity, boundaries, and contrasts between taste and flavour, plenty and scarcity, tradition and modernity, familiarity and novelty, the religious and the secular, the domesticated and the wild, satiety and hunger, continuity and change. The authors work within very different academic disciplines, come from different nations and speak different languages at home. Nevertheless, the variety of information provided in this volume has a general cohesion and no polemical disagreements. Of course, there are still many pieces missing from the jigsaw, which readers are challenged to fill in future research and publications.

References

Campbell, C. (1987) *The Romantic Ethic and the Spirit of Modern Consumerism*, Basil Blackwell, Oxford

Chapman, M. (1990) The framework for multidisciplinary perspectives on food, in M. Chapman and H.M. Macbeth (eds.), *Food for Humanity: Crossdisciplinary Readings*, Centre for the Sciences of Food and Nutrition, Oxford

Hladik, C.M. and Simmen, B. (1996) Taste perception and feeding behavior in nonhuman primates and human populations, *Evolutionary Anthropology*, 5:58-71.

James, A. (1979) Confections, concoctions and conceptions, *Journal of the Anthropological Society of Oxford*, 10(2): 83-95

James, A. (in press) How British is British food? A view from anthropology, in P. Caplan, (ed.) *Food, Identity and Health*, Routledge, London

Macbeth, H. (1989) Nature/nurture: the false dichotomies, *Anthropology Today*, 5(4): 12-15

Mintz, S. (1996) *Tasting Food, Tasting Freedom*, Beacon Press, Boston

Pilgrim, F.J. (1961) What foods do people accept or reject?, *Journal of the American Dietetic Association*, 38: 439-43

2. PRIMATE MODELS FOR TASTE AND FOOD PREFERENCES

Claude Marcel Hladik

In this chapter, a standard classification of taste qualities (salty, bitter, sour and sweet) is followed in order to present data on the taste perception of human populations and non-human primates. Of course, this classical form of presentation does not imply that we can still think about taste perception in terms of a simple correspondence between these different 'taste qualities' with the taste bud responses and their integration into the central system of perception. As explained by Edmund Rolls in this volume, the integration of taste qualities is determined by a complex neuronal network. And even when we consider the first contact of sapid substances with the taste buds of our tongue, each substance elicits responses from various categories of taste buds (Faurion, 1988) and never from a single class, as previously supposed, for example when tasting pure salt or pure acid. These stimuli result in a complex signal on the taste nerve, a kind of 'signature' characterising each sapid substance (Hladik and Simmen, 1997). Since the survival of most species may depend upon such signals, this discussion about primate models will be focused on the characteristics of these initial taste responses.

Salt Perception among the Inuit and Other Human Populations

The response to sodium chloride is one of these complex signals which is characterised as 'salty', a semantic taste descriptor (Faurion, 1993) common to most human populations. However, the Inuit people living on the eastern coast of Greenland have shown an extreme sensitivity to salt – as compared with the sensitivity found in any other population that has been tested. These results can be interpreted in terms of dietary adaptation of the Inuit to their particular environment.

Greenland is an immense icy desert, totally covered by an ice cap which reaches a thickness of four thousand metres; so, human settlements are limited to a narrow coastal fringe, along fjords, where the ice can melt during the summer months. On the other hand this coastal fringe is characterised by an extreme abundance of food resources, due to the high productivity of cold seas which have a high amount of dissolved carbon dioxide, thus more plankton than in warm seas, thus more fish, thus more seals. The Greenland coastal zone has been inhabited by humans for about four thousand years, first by palaeoeskimo populations, and now by the modern Inuit population (Robbe, 1994).

The staple food that provided – and still provides – most calories in the Inuit diet, is seal meat and fat, currently that of the ringed seal *(Pusa hispida)*. Young seals are caught with nets permanently set under the sea ice, or hunted from a small boat during the summer months. The seal meat is always boiled in water and not salted much. It is generally eaten and shared in a common dish, with several kin and affines, since sharing is one of the most important aspects of the Inuit way of life (Robbe, 1994). Thus this traditional life of hunter-gatherers, now integrated in a modern socioeconomic context, implies a diet with a particularly high protein content.

As a result, drinking large amounts of water is a physiological necessity, contributing to the elimination of urea that accumulates in the blood stream. The fact that all eskimo populations used to drink a remarkably high quantity of fresh water was noticed by the earlier explorers of Greenland, and more recently discussed by Draper (1977), who showed its importance as a feedback process without which the excess urea would not be properly eliminated. Furthermore, a diet that includes a high amount of protein induces a proportionally high dietary induced thermogenesis (DIT), which in turn fosters an increase of meat consumption to balance the calorie input/output. It is also a necessity to include fat (or a starchy staple, when available), together with meat, in the diet of hunter-gatherers, to minimise DIT and urea excretion (Speth, 1987).

During most of the year, drinking water had to be found by the Inuit in the form of freshwater ice, in the icebergs and iceblocks which had originated from the continental ice cap and become immobilised in the sea ice, near the coast during winter. This continental ice of blue-green colour used to be carefully chosen before being broken with an ice-pick and carried back home to be melted. The ice-collecting practice has recently vanished, since distribution of fresh water pumped under the ice of small lakes has been organised by elected authorities of the Inuit villages.

Figure 2.1 Taste thresholds for sodium chloride in different human populations and among non-human primate species.

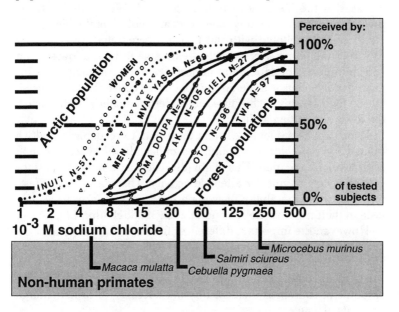

Top: Each curve shows, for a given population (or a group of populations), the cumulative percentages of people able to recognise the taste of a solution at the concentration indicated in millimoles on the horizontal axis.
(*Source:* Hladik et al., 1986)
Bottom: mean thresholds for non human primate species, on the same scale.
(*Source:* Glaser, 1986)

Nevertheless, the traditional quest for drinking water appears to be the most likely explanation for the results of tests on taste sensitivity to sodium chloride carried out among the Inuit population (Figure 2.1, Top). This argument is strengthened by comparative results obtained from various other populations of the world, for example from tests on Pygmies whose diet also includes a very high amount of protein. There is a remarkable and significant difference in taste sensitivity between the Inuit subjects, of whom fifty percent can identify as 'salty' a solution of sodium chloride diluted as low as eight millimoles, and most other populations for whom this median taste sensitivity is around forty millimoles; it reaches one hundred millimoles – that is 5.8 g per litre – for Pygmies. The extremely high sensitivity to sodium chloride of the Inuit population can be explained as the result of a selective pressure exerted during several centuries or millennia. As this population uses a large quantity of drinking water, found in a coastal environment, there is a risk of an excess of sodium intake (and the subsequent risk of cardiovascular diseases) if the ice is not carefully selected. When the ice to be melted for drinking water is taken from an iceblock embedded in sea ice, it can be polluted with salt that has penetrated by capillarity action or otherwise. Accordingly, being able to taste a low sodium concentration is of paramount importance to discriminate good ice from bad ice. This is done on the spot of ice collection and necessitates a high sensitivity, because the colder the material to be tasted, the lower the tasting ability.

It also appears (Figure 2.1) that the ability to recognise as salty a diluted sodium chloride solution is significantly more acute among Inuit women than men. This might just reflect a training effect, since collecting ice is typically a female activity. The results of our tests may just show the ability of women to identify quickly what they taste in their mouths (Robbe and Hladik, 1988; Hladik, 1995).

However, the important differences that were found between the Inuit and other populations cannot be explained in terms of training effect and are more likely to reflect the long-term adaptation of both sexes to an environment where the risk of ingesting excessive amounts of sodium is increased by the necessity of drinking large amounts of water.

Comparative Data on Salt Perception by Non-Human Primates

The comparison of these taste thresholds for sodium chloride with those of non-human primate species (Figure 2.1, Bottom) shows that interspecific variations are within the same range as those found among human populations.

Although the method for determining taste threshold is necessarily different for non-human primates, the values obtained from a two-bottle test (as described by Simmen in this volume) can be compared with the median values observed in human populations, because, in both cases, the recognition of the substance is necessary to elicit a recorded response. For human populations, the tests were conducted by presenting at random glucose, fructose, sucrose, sodium chloride, organic acids, and bitter substances, in the order of weakest solution to increasing concentrations. After rinsing with plain water these solutions were flushed on to the tongue in a standard amount (2 ml). Following this procedure (Hladik et al., 1986), obtained recognition thresholds for which a statistical test (chi square) had shown significant differences between human populations.

Under natural conditions, non-human primate populations are rarely exposed to high sodium intake; but the reactivity of the macaques to low sodium chloride solution could possibly reflect the adaptation of some populations to a coastal environment: there is unfortunately no record of the taste sensitivity of the crab-eating macaque.

Conversely, the possibility of a lack of sodium has been proposed by some authors to explain why some non-human primate species ingest pieces of termite mounds or other small amounts of earth (geophagy). This hypothesis was tested (Hladik and Viroben, 1974) by comparing the sodium content of earth samples with that of the whole diet (a mixture of fruits and leaves). In all instances, the sodium content of the natural diet was higher than the sodium available in the earth samples. Accordingly, geophagy was not considered as a way of finding sodium chloride in 'mineral foods' since sodium concentration in these is below most known primate thresholds. Our hypothesis to explain this ingestion of earth, mostly clay, is that this material can bind with the tannins, which are adsorbed on to the surface of clay particles, and thus neutralise the tannin content of the leaves ingested in large amounts at certain periods – precisely the periods during which geophagy was observed.

However, data on taste sensitivity to sodium are still relatively scarce for non-human primates. It will be more appropriate, therefore, to discuss the interspecific variation of taste responses in relation to other tasty substances for which ingestion or rejection can be a matter of survival.

Bitter and Acid Substances: Taste Sensitivity and Avoidance

Bitter substances and other natural products such as tannins and strong acids have a deterrent effect on food choices, with disgust at the origin of cultural preferences as discussed by Schiefenhövel in this volume. This behavioural response has been observed, even in newborn humans and newborn non-human primates (Steiner and Glaser, 1984). It is adaptive against the risk of being poisoned (many alkaloids, toxic or not, taste bitter). Various other plant products, the most abundant being tannins, may inhibit intestinal absorption when they bind to protein. The efficiency of the avoidance behaviours, therefore, can be enhanced by strategies such as geophagy, as mentioned above.

Figure 2.2 Taste thresholds for quinine hydrochloride in different human populations and among non-human primate species.

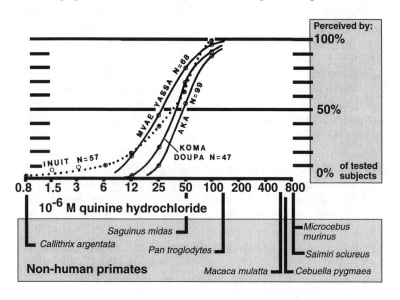

Top: Each curve shows, for a given population (or a group of populations), the cumulative percentages of people able to recognise the taste of a solution at the concentration indicated in micromoles on the horizontal axis. (*Source*: Hladik et al., 1986)
Bottom: mean thresholds for non human primate species, on the same scale. (*Source*: Glaser, 1986; Simmen, 1994)

The recognition thresholds of bitter substances in the various human populations so far tested (Figure 2.2, Top) are grouped in a very narrow range, in spite of the importance of inter-individual variation. The median threshold for quinine hydrochloride is about 25 micromoles (that is 0.009 g per litre) and there is no significant difference between the different populations. This high sensitivity to the bitter taste of quinine and other potentially harmful substances can be interpreted as the result of selective pressure, since human foraging populations, who lived inside or outside the tropical forests, have been faced with and are still facing the risk of being poisoned by ingesting such substances.

Some non-human primate species show a relatively low sensitivity to bitter substances and appear as more tolerant to bitter chemicals (Figure 2.2, Bottom). Here, again, it is important take into account the different methods used for testing humans and non-human primates. The recent results obtained by Simmen (1994) using a behavioural test (two-bottle test) on neotropical primate species, revealed contrasting differences between species that are closely related but have different dietary preferences. The extreme sensitivity of *Callithrix argentata* (0.8 micromole) can be opposed to the low sensitivity of the pygmy marmoset, *Cebuella pygmaea*, (threshold around six hundred micromoles). This last species obtains its staple food (gums and tree exudates) by biting and perforating the bark of various trees that may contain high amounts of chemicals such as quinine, which is found in the bark of the cinchona; accordingly its low reactivity to quinine is an adaptive response, but it is not necessarily in relation to a low taste sensitivity. In this case, the behavioural test yields results concerning avoidance threshold, that might be higher than the recognition threshold.

The recognition thresholds of acids are as low for humans as for non-human primates. For instance citric acid is recognised by human populations below four millimoles (Hladik et al., 1986) and elicits reactions in non-human primates between four and eight millimoles (Glaser, 1986). However, these reactions, generally of avoidance (e.g., at six millimoles for the pygmy marmoset) correspond to preferential choice, at least for one species, the Night Monkey, *Aotus trivirgatus*, (at four millimoles). Such ambiguous responses to a chemical which is widespread in both unripe and ripe fruits are not really surprising, since many foods and drinks appreciated by humans are a mixture of diluted acids with sweet tasting substances.

Sweet Preferences, Taste Threshold Variation and Supra-Threshold Responses

The positive side of taste perception is certainly as important, in terms of biological adaptation, as the negative responses of avoidance that are discussed above. For instance, the responses of non-human primate species to various sugars – presented in this volume by Simmen – play an essential role for balancing the energy input through food choices.

Figure 2.3 Taste thresholds for glucose and sucrose in different human populations and among non-human primate species.

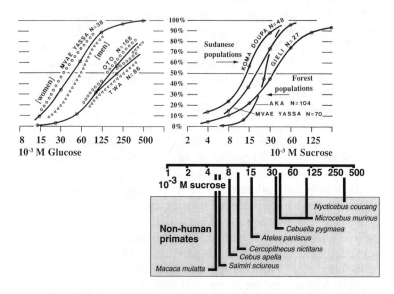

Top: Each of the curves shows, for a given population (or a group of populations), the cumulative percentages of people able to recognise the taste of a solution at the concentration indicated in millimoles on the horizontal axis.
(*Source:* Hladik et al., 1986)
Bottom: mean thresholds for non-human primate species, on the same scale.
(*Source:* Glaser, 1986; Simmen, this volume)

The comparison of taste thresholds of different human populations for different sugars (Figure 2.3, top) first revealed significant differences, especially when comparing the populations of the rain forest (e.g., Pygmies) with those living outside of the African forest (Hladik, 1993). The latter have a better sensitivity to glucose and sucrose, with a median taste threshold at ten millimoles for sucrose. Among the populations who have a low threshold for glucose (i.e., high sensitivity), a significant difference is found between taste sensitivity of men and of women. The latter always show a higher sensitivity, although this difference is not significant for Pygmies.

Some of these taste differences between population samples and taste differences between sexes can be explained by a learning effect, since the women are in charge of collecting wild food products and cooking. However, as in the case of the Inuit and their great acuity in tasting sodium chloride, when comparing forest populations and those living outside the forest who show a higher taste sensitivity to sugar, the most likely explanation of such differences is a long-term adaptive response of the taste system to the environment. Due to the coevolutionary history of animals and plants producing fleshy fruits, the African rain forest is extremely rich in fruits with a high sugar content (Hladik, 1993). Accordingly, the selective pressure for a higher sensitivity to sugar is likely to occur outside of the forest, where fruiting species are present in small number and have a relatively low sugar content.

The large range in taste sensitivity to sugar of non-human primates (Figure 2.3, Bottom) partly reflects this environmental initial condition. For instance, the pygmy marmoset *(Cebuella pygmaea)* has a rather high threshold for sucrose (above thirty millimoles), whereas the threshold of the Rhesus Monkey *(Macaca mulatta)*, which lives in open dry forests, is at five millimoles. These responses to sugars of non-human primates, recorded by Glaser (1986) and more recently by Simmen (this volume), are close to, and in some instances exactly the same as the physiological taste threshold, i.e., the minimum concentration eliciting a response on the taste nerve, the *chorda tympani.*

For one species, the Lesser Mouse Lemur *(Microcebus murinus)* there are two different thresholds shown in Figure 2.3. These two thresholds correspond to the seasonal variation of the taste response recorded by Simmen and Hladik (1988). It allows a kind of 'tuning' of the feeding behaviour of *M. murinus,* according to the food resources available during the drastic seasonal changes that occur in the forests of the west coast of Madagascar. In this case, we found that the physiological taste threshold does not show any significant variation (Hellekant et al., 1993). Accordingly, the variation of the taste response to sugar of *M. murinus* occurs at a higher level of taste perception, in the complex network of the taste signal processing, and results in a decreased motivation for sweet tasting substances.

Although seasonal variation is generally not as acute as that of the forests of Madagascar inhabited by *M. murinus,* it is widespread, even in the rain forest environment, affecting food availability for wild primates and for human populations (Hladik, 1988). Taste perception might be affected by these short-term changes. Nevertheless, taste threshold is only one important parameter influencing food choices. Sugar concentration in the pulp of most fruits available in the rain forest is ten to fifty times higher than the taste threshold of non-human primates and human populations (Hladik, 1993). Most food choices are obviously made at a concentration level well above the threshold.

The supra-threshold responses observed by Simmen (1992; this volume), and their various patterns among different species, can considerably increase motivation in relation to hedonic aspects of soluble substances. The increase of the hedonic dimension with sugar concentration (as measured by the increased consumption) is not the same in different species, for example when comparing fructose intake by frugivorous primates (e.g., *Callithrix argentata*) with that by species feeding mainly on gums and tree exudates (e.g., *Cebuella pygmaea*). Although their physiological aspects need further investigation, these profiles of the supra-threshold taste response help to explain why the different species maintain specific food choices, even when the environment can provide foods of similar composition.

Conclusion: Taste Responses and Food Choices

These various supra-threshold responses to sweet tasting substances can explain why frugivorous primates such as macaques and chimpanzees have sufficient motivation to obtain sugary fruits for them to be efficient foragers over extremely large territories, and are able to spot the most scattered plant species with the most nutritious fruits since these can provide the energy requirements of such large animals.

Positive responses are not limited to sugars and other sweet substances. For instance when the chimpanzees in Gabon 'fish' the *Ponerinae* ants by pushing and shaking a small twig inside the nest hole and pulling it out with one large ant biting it, there is a very special excitement in the group (Hladik, 1988). The chimpanzees, obviously, take great pleasure in cracking the ants under their teeth reducing them to a juice. This activity as a whole requires attention and skill and the reward must be adaptive. However, there is no sugar (or very little) in the ant juice, which mostly contains amino acids and peptones. Such substances, found in several animal prey, together with monosodium glutamate – the *umami* of the Japanese authors – can elicit the kind of taste responses analysed by Rolls (this volume), which corresponds to a high hedonic reward. There are several other soluble substances of similar interest in animal prey and food plants, especially in the juice of a liana stem, *Hypselodelphis violocea*, eaten throughout the year, and in the tiny leaf buds of a leguminous tree, *Baphia leptobotrys*, of which more than fifty percent of the dry weight is protein. The taste 'signature' of these substances and the associated supra-threshold response is a major part of an efficient adaptation to the diversity of the rain forest environment.

For humans, as for non-human primates, this great variety of chemicals which elicit negative and positive taste responses is still an open field for investigation. To study the progressive shaping of these responses in a young primate is probably the best way to understand the great distance from this purely biological perspective, which is relevant when considering the sociocultural aspects of the changes in food choices and preferences among humans.

References

Draper, H.H. (1977) The aboriginal Eskimo diet in modern perspective, *American Anthropologist*, 79: 303-16

Faurion, A. (1988) Naissance et obsolence du concept de quatre qualités en gustation, *Journal d'Agriculture Traditionelle et de Botanique Appliquée*, 35: 21-40

Faurion, A. (1993) Why four semantic taste descriptors and why only four? *11th International Conference on the Physiology of Food and Fluid Intake*, Oxford, July 1993, Abstract: 58

Glaser, D. (1986) Geschmacksforschung bei Primaten, *Vierteljahrsschrift der Naturforschenden Gesellschaft in Zürich*, 131: 92-110

Hellekant, G., Hladik, C.M., Dennys, V., Simmen, B., Roberts, T.W. and Glaser, D. (1993) On the relationship between sweet taste and seasonal body weight changes in a primate (*Microcebus murinus*). *Chemical Senses*, 18: 27-33

Hladik, C.M. (1988) Seasonal variation in food supply for wild primates, in I. de Garine and G.A. Harrison (eds.), *Coping with uncertainty in Food Supply,* Clarendon Press, Oxford: 1-25

Hladik, C.M. (1993) Fruits of the rain forest and taste perception as a result of evolutionary interactions, in C.M.Hladik, A. Hladik, O.F.Linares, A.Semple, M.Hadley (eds.), *Tropical Forests, People and Food: Biocultural Interactions and Applications to Development,* Unesco/Parthenon Publishing Group: 73-82

Hladik, C.M. (1995) Différenciation sexuelle du comportement alimentaire chez les Primates non humains et chez l'Homme, in A.Ducros and M.Panoff (eds.), *La Frontière des Sexes,* Presses Universitaires de France, Paris, 73-103

Hladik, C.M., Robbe, B. and Pagezy, H. (1986) Sensibilité gustative différentielle des populations Pygmées et non Pygmées de forêt dense, de Soudaniens et d'Eskimos, en rapport avec l'environnement biochimique, *C. R. Acad. Sc.* Paris, série III, 303: 453-8

Hladik, C.M. and Simmen, B. (1997) Taste perception and feeding behavior in nonhuman primates and human populations, *Evolutionary Anthropology*, 4: 161-74

Hladik, C.M. and Viroben, G. (1974) Géophagie et nutrition minérale chez les Primates sauvages, *C. R. Acad. Sc.*, Paris, série D, 279: 1,393-6

Robbe, B. and Hladik, C.M. (1988) Perception et consommation du sel dans la société Inuit de la côte orientale du Groenland, *Journal d'Agriculture Traditionelle et de Botanique Appliquée*, 35: 67-75

Robbe, P. (1994) *Les Inuit d'Ammassalik, Chasseurs de l'Arctique*, Mémoires du Muséum National d'Histoire Naturelle, T. 159: 389, Éditions du Muséum National d'Histoire Naturelle, Paris

Simmen, B. (1992) Seuil de discrimination et réponses supraliminaires à des solutions de fructose en fonction du régime alimentaire des primates Callitrichidae, *C.R. Acad. Sci.*, Paris, série III, 315: 151-7

Simmen, B. (1994) Taste discrimination and diet differentiation among New World primates, in D.J.Chivers and P.Langer (eds.), *The Digestive System of Mammals: Food, Form and Function*, Cambridge University Press, 150-65

Simmen, B. and Hladik, C.M. (1988) Seasonal variation of taste threshold for sucrose in a Prosimian species, *Microcebus murinus*, *Folia Primatologica*, 51: 152-7

Speth, J.D. (1987) Early hominid subsistence strategies in seasonal habitats, *Journal of Archaeological Sciences.*, 14: 13-29

Steiner, J.E. and Glaser, D. (1984) Differential behavioral responses to taste stimuli in non-human primates, *Journal of Human Evolution*, 13: 709-23

3. FOOD PREFERENCES IN NEOTROPICAL PRIMATES IN RELATION TO TASTE SENSITIVITY

Bruno Simmen

Introduction

The study of taste perception in non-human primates is of particular interest in understanding the biological and evolutionary basis of human feeding habits. Although taste perception is one of the first steps in assessing the quality of food, its functional role in the context of species adaptation to the biochemical environment has been little studied so far. Taste thresholds for various compounds may largely differ between primate species (Glaser, 1986; Hladik and Simmen, 1996), and we would expect, for instance, that there are some relationships between levels of taste discrimination and food choices. In this respect, research in a comparative perspective allows us to define to what extent phylogenetic constraints combine with the diversifying effects of adaptation (continuity versus changes) to shape the taste system. In order to determine whether interspecific differences of food choices may be sustained by differences of taste perception, it is necessary:

1. to study feeding strategies of wild primates with regard to the biochemical composition of foods, especially the water-soluble compounds which are likely to elicit taste sensations, and

2. to get an objective measure of species sensitivity.

This chapter presents results obtained on sympatric neotropical primates inhabiting the primary rain forest as well as a comparison of eco-ethological data with behaviour measured under experimental conditions in captivity. I shall mainly refer to taste discrimination and preference for soluble sugars which, among the different psychosensory aspects of the oropharyngeal stimulation, have been widely studied in primates.

Chemical Correlates of Primate Food Choices: a Case Study

Data presented here are part of a five-and-a-half month field study carried out in French Guiana during the rainy season which corresponds to a period of high fruit availability. The observations were initially made on red howler monkeys and black spider monkeys *(Alouatta seniculus and Ateles paniscus)* which are both arboreal primates weighing six to eight kilogrammes. It was particularly interesting to compare food choices between these related primates because, according to Kleiber's law, species having similar body weights are likely to have similar basal energy needs. The study was later extended to a smaller cebid monkey (about three kilogrammes), the capuchin monkey *Cebus apella.*

Based on the classical feeding frequency method (Struhsaker, 1975), estimates of diets show that spider and capuchin monkeys are mainly frugivores (> seventy-five percent of total feeding records) in contrast to howler monkeys which include a large proportion of young leaves (sixty-two percent of total feeding units) in addition to fruits in their diet. Furthermore, howler monkeys feed on immature fruits and old leaves, a pattern which is not observed in the former species. As pointed out by many field workers, frugivory and folivory correspond to distinct feeding strategies adjusted to the differential biomass of leaves and fruits. Frugivorous primates such as spider and capuchin monkeys have larger home ranges, longer daily travel distances and spend more time moving and feeding than sympatric folivores such as howler monkeys which can find leaves over small territories. This is also directly connected with morphological and physiological specialisations of the digestive tract (Chivers and Hladik, 1980). Howler monkeys are hindgut fermenters, that is their caecum is capacious and food transit time is about sixteen to thirty hours (Milton, 1984). This allows them to obtain a large part of their energy and proteins from cellulose and hemicellulose of leaves which require fermentation processes and symbiotic associations with bacteria. Given that ripe fruits are usually characterised by high metabolisable energy but low protein contents as compared with young leaves (Table 3.1), species feeding predominantly on fruits have various possibilities for meeting their protein requirements. Digestive tracts of spider and capuchin monkeys are relatively simple and transit time is much shorter (three to eight hours according to Milton, 1984). Spider monkeys may be considered as fruit specialists because they compensate for the low nitrogen content of fruit by ingesting large amounts of pulp, to which they add only low proportions of young leaves. The small body size of capuchin monkeys makes predation on invertebrates, which provide an important additional source of nitrogen, more advantageous.

Table 3.1 Nutrient composition of foods eaten by primates in French Guiana.

	Water	Protein	Lipids	Soluble Sugars
	% range (mean)	%dry weight range (mean)		
Young leaves	73.8-92.8 (83.6; n=7)	9.3-36.8 (21.5; n=7)	0.9-3.1 (1.7; n=6)	3.0-8.9 (4.6; n=6)
Ripe fruits	59.4-85.6 (76.1; n=13)	3.7-10.9 (6.3; n=9)	(49*) (n=1)	14.6-66.9 (41.7; n=8)
Nectar (*Norantea*)	90.0	0.1	n.d.	93

Together with digestive capabilities and long-term metabolic effects of foods, oropharyngeal factors also contribute to the adjustment of feeding behaviour to the biochemical environment. The fleshy part of most tropical fruits selected by primates is often scanty but is very sweet, and rich in soluble sugars. Differences in the content of water-soluble compounds between leaves and fruits (Table 3.2) suggest that howler monkey food choices are less influenced by sweet stimuli than those of spider and capuchin monkeys. This would explain, for instance, why sweet nectars of *Norantea* flowers are largely consumed by all primates with the exception of howler monkeys, although the liana bearing these flowers lies over trees normally entered by howler groups. There are several other plant species bearing fruits with high sugar content which are only eaten by spider and capuchin monkeys although these plants are available throughout territories of howler monkeys.

Table 3.2 Water-soluble compounds of some important foods eaten by primates.

	Soluble content (SC)	Protein in SC	Sugars in SC
	% total dry weight range (mean)	% of SC dry weight range (mean)	
Young leaves	17.2-39.7 (27.8; n=5)	<0.5 (n=2)	10.6-29.9 (18.0; n=4)
Ripe fruits	22.6-85.0 (54.6; n=13)	0.1-4.7 (1.5; n=7)	27.6-90.6 (67.8; n=8)
Nectar (*Norantea*)	100	0.1	93

A test of the hypothesis originally formulated by Marcel Hladik (1981), according to which frugivorous strategies are associated with a high efficiency of sweet stimulations, may be performed by recording taste responses to sugars in species exhibiting distinct dietary adaptations.

Comparative Aspects of Taste Discrimination of Carbohydrates

Taste thresholds are at present the only available parameters which have been extensively studied in primates but recent works (Simmen, 1992; 1994) have stressed the importance of characterising ingestive responses to supra-threshold concentrations of tastant. Indeed they appear to reflect the intensity of sweet stimuli and are thus particularly relevant to the question of how primates cope with the variation of sugar concentrations according to plant species and stage of ripeness. Both aspects will now be examined.

In several cases, taste thresholds determined by the behavioural procedure of the 'two-bottle test' have proven to be similar to values obtained using electrophysiological methods (Glaser and Hellekant, 1977; Ogawa et al., 1972). The 'two-bottle test' is thus a reliable method and involves long-term experiments in which the gustatory solution is presented simultaneously with tap water to the animals. The different concentrations are varied at random on a daily basis and taste threshold is considered as the lowest concentration for which the mean difference between the intake of solution and the intake of tap water differs significantly with a paired-sample t-test. For instance, in the case of *Cebus apella*, sucrose concentrations lower than 5 to 11 millimoles (mM) do not yield significant differences (P>0.5; Figure 3.1).

Figure 3.1 Results of the two-bottle test (sucrose) in *Cebus apella*.

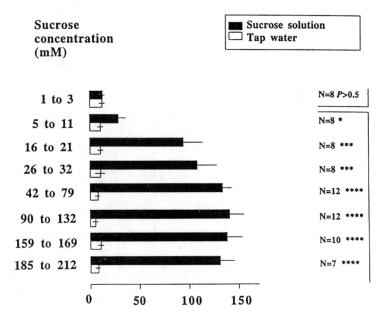

Liquid consumption in each test (ml)

*   p<0.05
***   p<0.01
****   p<0.001

As expected, the comparison of ecological data and taste thresholds for sucrose (Table 3.3) would indicate some relationship between feeding strategies and taste discrimination. Spider and capuchin monkeys exhibit the highest fruit diversities and longest daily travel distances, which reflect strategies of high energy input/ high energy costs, and their taste thresholds are amongst the lowest values that have been found so far in primates. Although this would support the hypothesis that motivation for fruit seeking is partly sustained by high palatability of soluble sugars, the picture is actually

Table 3.3 Aspects of feeding strategies and taste discrimination of sucrose in some neotropical primates.

	Number of fruit-flower species in the diet	Daily travel distance mean (range) m	**Taste threshold for sucrose** mM (this study)	References
French Guiana and Suriname				
Alouatta seniculus	97-35	700 (235-1,760)	n.d.	Julliot, 1992 (19 months)
Ateles paniscus	171-33	-(500-5,000)	16 ± 5	Van Roosmalen 1980 (26 months)
Cebus apella	135-5	2,300 (1,700-3,500)	8 ± 3	Zhang, 1994 (19 months)
Sanguinus midas	n.d.	n.d.	66[a]	
Peru				
Ateles paniscus	n.d.	1,977 (465-4,070)		Symington, 1988 (21 months)
Cebus apella	>130-2	2,100 (1,600-2,600)		Terborgh, 1983 (4 yrs) Janson et at., 1986 (>1 yr) Robinson & Janson, 1987 (>1 yr)
Saimiri sciureus	>90-2		6[a]	Terborgh, 1983 (4 yrs)
Saguinus fuscicollis	>32-2	1,200	50[a]	Terborgh, 1983 (4 yrs) Terborgh & Stern, 1987
Saguinus imperator	>31-3	1,400	n.d.	Terborgh, 1983 (4 yrs)

Notes: 1. Glaser (1986)
   2. The common names of primate genera are as follows:
      Alouatta = howlers; *Cebus* = capuchin monkeys; *Saimiri* = squirrel monkeys; *Saguinus* = tamarins

more complex than assumed here. For instance, it is not obvious to what extent differences of sugar palatability between frugivorous species actually affect the separation of dietary niches because many of the fleshy fruits with high soluble content are simultaneously and heavily utilised by several of these primates. Conversely, some plant species bearing sugar-rich fruits may not be utilised by all primates, but this is often in relation to factors other than taste. For instance, within *Sapotaceae* – one of the plant family most heavily used by primates at the study site – fruits have very similar chemical characteristics as regards sugar content (Simmen, 1991). They only differ in size, which is obviously an important factor when we bear in mind that primates ranging from five hundred grammes, such as tamarins *(Saguinus),* to eight kilogrammes must swallow the seeds to which pulp tightly adheres.

Figure 3.2 Taste thresholds for fructose in *Callitrichidae* and *Callimiconidae.*

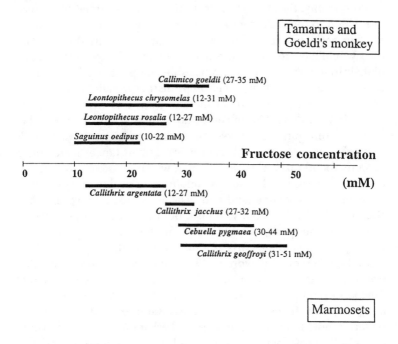

Top: Tamarins *(Saguinus),* Lion Tamarins *(Leontopitheus)* and Goeldi's monkey *(Callimico).*
Bottom: Marmosets *(Callithrix)* and Pigmy Marmoset *(Cebuella).*

Taste thresholds for sugars might also reflect phylogeny as indicated by similar values obtained in closely related species whatever their dietary tendencies (Simmen, et al., 1995). This occurs in prosimians (e.g., *Lemuridae, Cheirogalidae*) as well as in simians (e.g., *Cercopithecidae*). For instance, bamboo lemurs *Hapalemur griseus* and *Hapalemur simus* show high sensitivity to sugars, as in other frugivorous leumurids (Bonnaire and Simmen, 1994) although they appear to subsist on soluble sugar-poor diets (Glander et al., 1989). Similarly, within *Callitrichidae*, all species have largely overlapping taste thresholds for fructose within the range 10 to 51mM although some specialise on gums, which mainly contain polymerised sugars, and

some feed predominantly on fruits and nectars as regards the plant
part of their diets (Figure 3.2; Simmen, 1992). Contrasting with
responses to carbohydrates, taste thresholds for quinine hydrochloride are highly differentiated in these New World primates (Simmen,
1994). They reflect distinct levels of sensory and metabolic tolerance
to bitter secondary compounds which act as chemical defences
against herbivorous consumers.

Presumably, the ability to detect soluble sugars primarily evolved
in relation to the shift from insectivorous toward more frugivorous
diets in early primates. Species which later specialised on fibrous
diets would have retained taste sensitivity toward sugars close to that
of their frugivorous ancestors. A possible interpretation for the maintenance of high sensitivity levels in primates specialised on polysaccharides is that most of them include fruits and nectars to some
extent in their diets. This of course does not preclude the possibility
that leaf and gum eaters select their preferred non-sweet foods
through other sensory characteristics. For instance, it has been
recently found that a glucose polymer, which is tasteless to humans,
elicits a preferred and probably unique taste quality in rats as well
as in macaques (Sunderland and Sclafani, 1988; Giza et al., 1991;
Ramirez, 1991). The ability to taste both hexoses and polysaccharides might thus partly account for dietary flexibility in species using
non-reproductive plant parts as a main source of energy, but which
can adapt to more frugivorous diets according to food availability
(for instance gummivorous marmosets). In the opposite case, loss of
function would probably have resulted in low, or lack of, sensitivity,
as observed in felids and insectivores (Ramirez, 1990), but such a
pattern is not found in primates tested. Perhaps low sensitivity would
occur in the most folivorous primates, but there is at present no data
available on such species.

In fact affective perception of taste stimuli may be more relevant
than taste thresholds to the study of psychophysiological factors influencing feeding behaviour. It is not easy to discover what an animal
likes but recent results (Simmen, 1992) have demonstrated that closely
related species are better differentiated according to their responses to
supra-threshold concentrations of fructose than according to their dis-
criminative abilities. Although these ingestive responses may involve
metabolic effects, they nevertheless partly reflect the differential
palatability of sugars between species. Again the example is taken
from Callitrichidae. Although taste thresholds overlap in the nine
species tested (see above), rates of consumption for concentrations up
to 100 mM were lower in the most gummivorous marmosets *(Cebuella*
and *Callithrix jacchus)* than in frugivorous tamarins *(Saguinus, Leontop-*

ithecus spp. and *Callimico*, Simmen, 1992). Low palatability of fructose in the pygmy marmoset, *Cebuella pygmaea*, is consistent with the observation that in the wild, some populations feed on a few exudate sources and do not include fruits in their diet. Accordingly, interspecific differences in the hedonic value of taste stimuli probably have large consequences on the selectivity of feeding behaviour.

Conclusion

Results presented in this chapter clearly indicate that a distinction must be made between the ability to detect sugars and the hedonic value of gustatory stimuli, in defining more precisely the role of taste in the feeding behaviour of primates. Although taste thresholds for sugars have potential implications for the detection of energy, the sensory reward produced by sugars may largely affect the occupation of specific feeding niches. Since species may share similar taste thresholds irrespective of dietary tendencies, it is now more important to determine whether the affective value of sweet stimuli is lower in primates feeding on leaves or gums than in those which are frugivorous/nectarivorous.

References

Bonnaire, L. and Simmen, B. (1994) Taste perception of fructose solutions and diet in lemuridae, *Folia Primatologica,* 63: 171-6

Chivers, D.J. and Hladik C.M. (1980) Morphology of the gastrointestinal tract in Primates: comparisons with other mammals in relation to diet, *Journal of Morphology,* 166: 337-86

Giza, B.K., Scott, T.R., Sclafani, A. and Antonucci, R.F. (1991) Polysaccharides as taste stimuli: their effect in the nucleus tractus solitarius of the rat, *Brain Research,* 555: 1-9

Glander, K.E., Wright, P.C., Seigler, D.S., Randrianasolo, V. and Randrianasolo B. (1989) Consumption of cyanogenic bamboo by a newly discovered species of bamboo lemur, *American Journal of Primatology,* 19: 119-24

Glaser, D. (1986) Geschmacksforschung bei Primaten, *Sonderdruck aus der Vierteljahrsschrift der Naturforschenden Gesellschaft in Zürich,* 131: 92-110

Glaser, D. and Hellekant G. (1977) Verhaltens und electrophysiologische Experimente über den Geschmackssinn bei *Saguinus midas tamarin* (Callitrichidae), *Folia Primatologica*, 28: 43-51

Hladik, C.M. (1981) Diet and the evolution of feeding strategies among forest Primates, in R.S.O. Harding and G. Teleki (eds.), *Omnivorous Primates: Gathering and Hunting in Human Evolution*, Columbia University Press, New York, R.S.O., 215-54

Hladik, C.M. and Simmen, B. (1996) Taste perception and feeding behavior in nonhuman primates and human populations, *Evolutionary Anthropology*, 5: 58-71

Hladik, C.M., Hladik, A., Bousset, J., Valdebouze, P., Viroben, G. and Delort-Laval J. (1971) Le régime alimentaire des primates de l'île de Barro Colorado (Panama), *Folia Primatologica*, 16: 85-122

Janson, C.H., Stiles, E.W. and D.H. White (1986) Selection on plant fruiting traits by brown capuchin monkeys: a multivariate approach, in A. Estrada and T. H. Fleming (eds.), *Frugivores and Seed Dispersal*, Dr. W. Junk Publishers, Dordrecht, 83-92

Julliot, C. (1992) *Utilisation des ressources alimentaires par le singe hurleur roux, Alouatta seniculus (Atelidae, Primates), en Guyane: impact de la dissémination des graines sur la régénération forestière*, Thèse de Doctorat de l'Université de Tours

Milton, K. (1984) The role of food-processing factors in primate food choice, in P.S. Rodman and J.G.H. Cant (eds.), *Adaptations for Foraging in Nonhuman Primates. Contributions to an Organismal Biology of Prosimians, Monkeys, and Apes*, Columbia University Press, New York, 249-79

Ogawa, H., Yamashita, S., Noma, A. and Sato M. (1972) Taste responses in the macaque monkey chorda tympani, *Physiology and Behavior*, 9: 325-331

Ramirez, I. (1990) Why do sugars taste good? *Neuroscience and Biobehavioral Reviews*, 14: 125-34

Ramirez, I. (1991) Does starch taste like polycose? *Physiology and Behavior*, 50: 389-92

Robinson, J.G. and C.H. Janson (1987) Capuchins, squirrel monkeys and atelines: socioecological convergence with Old World Monkeys, in B.B. Smuts, D.L. Cheney, R.M. Seyfarth, R.W. Wrangham and T.T. Struhsaker (eds.), *Primate Societies,* University of Chicago Press, 69-82

van Roosmalen, M.G.M. (1980) *Habitat preference, diet, feeding strategy and social organisation of the black spider monkey (Ateles paniscus paniscus Linnaeus 1758) in Surinam*, Ph.D., Agricultural University of Wageningen, Leersum

Simmen, B. (1991) *Stratégies alimentaires des primates néotropicaux en fonction de la perception des produits de l'environnement*, Thèse de Doctorat de l'Université Paris XIII, Villetaneuse

Simmen, B. (1992) Seuil de discrimination et réponses supraliminaires à des solutions de fructose en fonction du régime des primates Callitrichidae, *Comptes Rendus de l'Académie des Sciences de Paris*, 315: 151-7

Simmen, B. (1994) Taste discrimination and diet differentiation among New World primates, in D.J. Chivers and P. Langer (eds.), *The Digestive System in Mammals: Food, Form and Function*, Cambridge University Press, 150-65

Simmen, B., Hladik, C.M. and Martin, R.D (1995) Sweet and bitter taste discrimination and energy requirements in nonhuman primates, *Chemical Senses*, 20: 153 (abstract)

Struhsaker, T.T. (1975) *The Red Colobus Monkey*, University of Chicago Press

Sunderland, G. and Sclafani A. (1988) Taste preferences of squirrel monkeys and bonnet macaques for polycose, maltose and sucrose, *Physiology and Behavior*, 43: 685-90

Symington, M.M. (1988) Demography, ranging patterns, and activity budgets of black spider monkeys *(Ateles paniscus chamek)* in the Manu National Park, Peru, *American Journal of Primatology*, 15: 45-67

Terborgh, J. (1983) *Five New World Primates: A Study in Comparative Ecology*, Princeton University Press

Terborgh, J. and M. Stern (1987) The surreptitious life of the saddle-backed tamarin, *American Scientist*, 75: 260-9

4. NEURAL PROCESSING UNDERLYING FOOD SELECTION

Edmund T. Rolls

Introduction

Investigations of how the brain processes taste and olfactory stimuli and controls food intake have led to advances in our understanding of how food preferences are controlled. These are described in this chapter. More comprehensive treatments of the neural mechanisms of food intake control, and of olfactory and taste processing, are provided elsewhere (Rolls, 1989, 1993, 1994, 1995, 1996). The majority of the studies described were performed with monkeys *(Macaca mulatta or Macaca fascicularis),* as studies in these non-human primates are especially relevant to understanding processing and its disorders in the taste, olfactory, and food intake control systems, in humans.

Neuronal Activity in the Lateral Hypothalamus during Feeding

The lateral hypothalamus, located at the base of the brain (see Figure 4.1) is essential for the normal regulation of food intake, in that damage to it reduces eating, and impairs food intake control. To analyse what signals reach the hypothalamus, and the way in which it is involved in appetite, recordings have been made from single neurons (brain cells) in the lateral hypothalamus. It has been shown that there is a population of neurons in the lateral hypothalamus and substantia innominata of the monkey with responses which are related to feeding (see Rolls, 1993, 1994). These neurons, which comprised 13.6 percent in one sample of 764 hypothalamic neurons, respond to the taste and/or sight of food. Thus signals which are relevant to appetite, food selection, and the control of feeding, do reach the lateral hypothalamus.

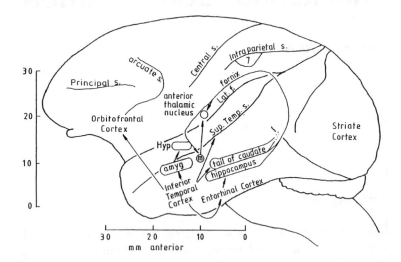

Figure 4.1 Some of the pathways described in the text are shown on this lateral view of the brain of the macaque monkey. amyg = amygdala; central s = central sulcus; Hyp = hypothalamus / substantia innominata / basal forebrain; Lat f = lateral (or Sylvian) fissure; m = mammillary body; Sup Temp s = superior temporal sulcus; 7 = posterior parietal cortex, area 7. The secondary taste and the primary olfactory cortex are within the orbitofrontal cortex. The secondary taste cortex and the primary olfactory cortex are just behind this.

Sensory-specific modulation of the responsiveness of lateral hypothalamic neurons

It has been shown that these lateral hypothalamic neurons respond to the sight and/or taste of a food only if the monkey has an appetite for that food. This was discovered in experiments in which the monkey was fed to satiety on one food, and the neuron stopped responding to that food, but did still respond to another food on which the

monkey had not been fed. Corresponding to this neuronal specificity of the effects of feeding to satiety, it was found that the monkey rejected the food on which he had been fed to satiety, but
accepted other foods which he had not been fed. These neurons
appear to be part of a food reward system in the lateral hypothalamus, in which hunger signals alter the reward value of the taste,
sight and smell of food, and thus contribute to the control of food
intake (Rolls, 1993, 1994).

Sensory-specific Satiety as a Determinant of Food Preferences in Humans

As a result of these neurophysiological and behavioural observations showing the specificity of satiety in the monkey, experiments
were performed to determine whether satiety was specific to foods
eaten in humans. It was found that the pleasantness of the taste of
food eaten to satiety decreased more than for foods that had not
been eaten (Rolls, Rolls et al., 1981). One implication of this finding
is that if one food is eaten to satiety, appetite reduction for other
foods is often incomplete, and this should mean that in humans too
at least some of the other foods will be eaten. This has been confirmed in an experiment in which either sausages or cheese with
crackers were eaten for lunch. The liking for the food eaten decreased
more than for the food not eaten and, when an unexpected second
course was offered, more was eaten if a subject had not been given
that food in the first course than if he had been given that food in the
first course (ninety-eight percent vs. forty percent of the first course
intake eaten in the second courses, p<0.01, Rolls et al., 1981). A further implication of these findings is that if a variety of foods is available, the total amount consumed will be more than when only one
food is offered repeatedly. This prediction has been confirmed in a
study in which humans ate more when offered a variety of sandwich
fillings than one filling or a variety of types of yoghurt which differed
in taste, texture and color. It has also been confirmed in a study in
which humans were offered a relatively normal meal of four courses,
and it was found that the change of food at each course significantly
enhanced intake (Rolls et al., 1984). As sensory factors such as similarity of colour, shape, flavour and texture are usually more important than metabolic equivalence in terms of protein, carbohydrate
and fat content in influencing how foods interact in this type of satiety, it has been termed 'sensory-specific satiety' (Rolls et al., 1982;
Rolls et al., 1981). It should be noted that this effect is distinct from

alliesthesia, in that alliesthesia is a change in the pleasantness of sensory inputs produced by internal signals (such as glucose in the gut) (see Cabanac, 1971), whereas sensory-specific satiety is a change in the pleasantness of sensory inputs which is accounted for at least partly by the external sensory stimulation received (such as the taste of a particular food), in that as shown above it is at least partly specific to the external sensory stimulation received.

The parallel between these studies of feeding in humans and of the neurophysiology of hypothalamic neurons in the monkey has been extended by the observation that in humans, sensory-specific satiety occurs for the sight as well as for the taste of food (Rolls et al., 1982). Further, to complement the finding that in the hypothalamus neurons are found which respond differently to food and to water (E.T. Rolls and colleagues, unpublished observations), and that satiety with water can decrease the responsiveness of hypothalamic neurons which respond to water, it has been shown that in humans motivation-specific satiety can also be detected. For example, satiety with water decreases the pleasantness of the sight and taste of water but not of food (Rolls, Rolls and Rowe, 1983).

The enhanced eating when a variety of foods is available, as a result of the operation of sensory-specific satiety, may have been advantageous in evolution in ensuring that different foods with important different nutrients were consumed, but today in humans, when a wide variety of foods is readily available, it may be a factor which can lead to overeating and obesity. In a test of this in the rat, it has been found that variety itself can lead to obesity (Rolls, Van Duijenvoorde and Rowe, 1983; see further Rolls and Hetherington, 1989).

Advances in understanding the neurophysiological mechanisms of sensory-specific satiety are being made in analyses of information processing in the taste and olfactory systems, as described below.

In addition to the sensory-specific satiety described above which operates primarily within (see above) and in the post-meal period (Rolls et al., 1984), there is now evidence for a long-term form of sensory-specific satiety (Rolls and de Waal, 1985). This was shown in a study in an Ethiopian refugee camp, in which it was found that refugees who had been in the camp for six months found the taste of their three regular foods less pleasant than that of three comparable foods which they had not been eating. The effect was a long-term form of sensory-specific satiety in that it was not found in refugees who had been in the camp and eaten the regular foods for only two days (Rolls and de Waal, 1985). It is suggested that it is important to recognise the operation of long-term sensory-specific satiety in conditions such as these, for it may enhance malnutrition if the regular foods become less acceptable and so are rejected, exchanged for other less nutritionally effective foods or goods, or inadequately prepared. It may be advantageous under these circumstances to attempt to minimise the operation of long-term sensory-specific satiety by providing some variety, perhaps even with spices (Rolls and de Waal, 1985). It is likely that such long-term sensory-specific satiety effects are more evident with foods with strong flavours than with foods which have bland flavours, such as most staple foods.

Learned Associations Between the Sight and Taste of Food

The responses of the hypothalamic neurons become associated with the sight of food as a result of learning (Mora et al., 1976; Wilson and Rolls, 1990). This type of learning is important for it allows organisms to respond appropriately to environmental stimuli which previous experience has shown to be foods. The brain mechanisms for this type of associative learning are in the amygdala and orbitofrontal cortex, as shown by the findings that lesions to these brain regions (see Figures 4.1 and 4.2) make food selection much less precise, impair learning associations between the sight of objects and their taste, and that neurons in these regions alter the visual stimuli to which they respond during visual-to-taste association learning (see Rolls, 1993, 1994, 1996).

Activity in the Gustatory Pathways during Feeding, and the Computation of Sensory-specific Satiety

The lateral hypothalamus has neuronal responses which are related to sensory-specific satiety, but the actual computation appears to be performed in the secondary taste cortex, through which taste signals reach the hypothalamus in primates (see Figures 4.1 and 4.2). The primary taste cortex is the first cortical area concerned with taste. It receives its taste inputs from the taste part of the thalamus. The secondary taste cortex is the second cortical processing area concerned with taste, and receives its taste inputs from the primary taste cortex (see Rolls, 1994, 1995).

Neurophysiological investigations have shown that in primates, the first stage in the taste system at which satiety influences processing is the secondary taste cortex, which forms part of the orbitofrontal cortex. Neurons also become more sharply tuned to individual tastants in

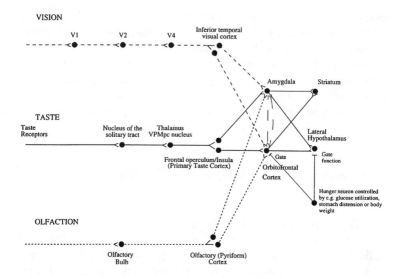

Figure 4.2 Schematic diagram showing some of the gustatory, olfactory, and visual pathways involved in processing sensory stimuli involved in the control of food intake. The secondary taste cortex, and the secondary olfactory cortex, are within the orbitofrontal cortex.

this region (Rolls, 1994). In addition to representations of the 'proto-typical' stimuli sweet, salt, bitter and sour, different neurons in this region respond to *umami* (protein) taste (e.g., glutamate, Baylis and Rolls, 1991), to astringent taste (as exemplified by tannic acid, and which is important in primate food selection, Critchley and Rolls, 1996b), and to a wide range of complex foods (Baylis and Rolls, in preparation). Thus it appears that the reduced acceptance of food as satiety develops, and the reduction in its pleasantness, are not pro-duced in primates by a reduction in the responses to gustatory stimuli of neurons in early taste processing in the brainstem (the nucleus of the solitary tract, see Figure 4.2), nor in the primary taste cortex (located in the frontal operculum and insula). (As described above, the responses of gustatory neurons in these areas do not decrease as sati-ety develops.) Indeed, after feeding to satiety, humans reported that the taste of the food on which they had been satiated tasted almost as intense as when they were hungry, though much less pleasant (Rolls, Rolls and Rowe, 1983). This comparison is consistent with the possi-bility that activity in the primary taste cortex as well as the brainstem (nucleus of the solitary tract) does not reflect the pleasantness of the

taste of a food, but rather its sensory qualities independently of motivational state. On the other hand, the responses of the neurons in the
orbitofrontal taste area (which includes the secondary taste cortex)
and in the lateral hypothalamus are modulated by satiety, and it is
presumably in areas such as these that neuronal activity may be
related to whether a food tastes pleasant, and to whether the human
or animal will work to obtain and then eat the food, that is to say
whether the food is rewarding.

These results provide evidence on the nature of the mechanisms
which underlie sensory-specific satiety. The results suggest that such
sensory-specific satiety cannot be largely accounted for by adaptation
at the receptor level, nor in the brainstem, nor in the primary taste
cortex, to the food which has been eaten to satiety, otherwise modulation of neuronal responsiveness should have been apparent in the
recordings made in these regions. Indeed, the findings suggest that
sensory-specific satiety is not represented in the primary gustatory
cortex. It is thus of particular interest that a decrease in the response
of orbitofrontal cortex neurons occurs which is partly specific to the
food which has just been eaten to satiety (Rolls et al., 1989).

These findings lead to the following proposed neuronal mechanism for sensory-specific satiety. The tuning of neurons becomes
more specific for gustatory stimuli through the brainstem (nucleus of
the solitary tract), gustatory thalamus, and primary taste cortex (see
Figure 4.2). Satiety, habituation and adaptation are not features of
the responses in these processing stages. The tuning of neurons
becomes even more specific in the orbitofrontal cortex, but here
there is some effect of satiety by internal signals such as gastric dis-
tension and glucose utilisation, and in addition habituation with a
time course of several minutes which lasts for one to two hours is a
feature of the synapses which are activated. Owing to the relative
specificity of the tuning of orbitofrontal taste neurons, this results in
a decrease in the response to that food, but different foods continue
to activate other neurons. (For orbitofrontal cortex neurons that
respond to two similar tastes before satiety, it is suggested that the
habituation which results in a loss of the response to the taste of the
item eaten to satiety occurs because of habituation of the afferent
neurons or synapses on to these orbitofrontal cortex neurons.) Then,
the orbitofrontal cortex neurons have the required response properties, and it is only then necessary for other parts of the brain to use
the activity of the orbitofrontal cortex neurons to reflect the reward
value of that particular taste.

It is suggested that the computational significance of this architecture is as follows (see also Rolls, 1989). If satiety were to operate at

an early level of sensory analysis, then because of the broadness of tuning of neurons, responses to non-foods would become attenuated as well as responses to foods (and this could well be dangerous if poisonous non-foods became undetectable). This argument becomes even more compelling when it is realised that satiety typically shows some specificity for the particular food eaten, with others not eaten in the meal remaining relatively pleasant (see above). Unless tuning were relatively fine, this mechanism could not operate, for reduction in neuronal firing after one food had been eaten would inevitably reduce behavioural responsiveness to other foods. Indeed, it is of interest to note that such a sensory-specific satiety mechanism can be built by arranging for tuning to particular foods to become relatively specific at one level of the nervous system (as a result of categorisation processing in earlier stages), and then at this stage (but not at prior stages) to allow habituation to be a property of the synapses, as proposed above.

Thus information processing in the taste system illustrates an important principle of higher nervous system function in primates, namely that it is only after several or many stages of sensory information processing (which produce efficient categorisation of the stimulus) that there is an interface to motivational systems, to other modalities, or to systems involved in association memory (Rolls and Treves, 1997).

Convergence between Taste and Olfactory Processing to Represent Flavour

At some stage in taste processing, it is likely that taste representations are brought together with inputs from different modalities, for example with olfactory inputs to form a representation of flavour. Takagi and his colleagues (see Takagi, 1991) have found an olfactory area in the medial orbitofrontal cortex. In the posterior orbitofrontal cortex is the area investigated by Thorpe et al. (1983) in which are found many neurons with visual and some with gustatory responses. In a recent investigation of the caudolateral orbitofrontal cortex taste area (Rolls, 1989; Rolls and Baylis, 1994), we found that of the single neurons which responded to any of these modalities, many were unimodal (taste forty-seven percent, olfactory twelve percent, visual ten percent), but were found in close proximity to each other. Some single neurons showed convergence, responding for example to taste and visual inputs (seventeen percent), taste and olfactory inputs (ten percent), and olfactory and visual inputs (four percent). Some of these multimodal single neurons had corresponding sensitivities in the two modalities, in that they responded best to sweet tastes (e.g., 1M glucose), and responded more in a visual discrimination task to the visual stimulus which signified sweet fruit juice than to that which signified saline; or responded to sweet taste, and in an olfactory discrimination task to fruit odour. The different types of neurons (unimodal in different modalities, and multimodal) were frequently found close to one another in tracks made into this region, consistent with the hypothesis that the multimodal representations are actually being formed from unimodal inputs to this region. Consistent with this, in recent experiments E.T. Rolls and H. Critchley (see Rolls, 1996) have shown that the responses of some neurons in this region to an odour can be altered when the taste with which the odour is associated is altered in an olfactory discrimination task. Further evidence linking these olfactory neurons to the control of responses to food is that we (Critchley and Rolls, 1996a) have found that the responses of these olfactory neurons decrease selectively for the odour of a food with which the monkey is fed to satiety. Thus the responses of at least some of these neurons are related to sensory-specific satiety effects for odour. Olfactory sensory-specific satiety is a feature of human feeding behaviour (Rolls and Rolls, 1997) which is involved in food selection. These results show that there are regions in the orbitofrontal cortex of primates where the sensory modalities of taste and olfaction converge; that in many cases the neurons have corresponding sensitivities across modalities; and that the neurons have responses which are related to motivation, in that they are related to sensory-specific satiety. This may be the part of the primate nervous system where flavour is computed. In addition, information about the texture of food also influences neurons in this region.

Consistent with these neurophysiological studies, food preferences are disrupted by damage to the orbitofrontal cortex, in that monkeys with damage to the orbitofrontal cortex select and eat foods which are normally rejected (Butter et al., 1969; Baylis and Gaffan, 1991). Their food choice behaviour is very similar to that of monkeys with amygdala lesions (Baylis and Gaffan, 1991). Lesions of the orbitofrontal cortex also lead to a failure to correct feeding responses when these become inappropriate (see Rolls, 1993, 1994, 1996).

The convergence of visual information on to neurons in this region not only allows associations to be learned between the sight of a food and its taste and smell, but also may provide the neural basis for the well-known effect which the sight of a food has on its perceived taste.

Functions of the Amygdala and Temporal Cortes in Feeding

Bilateral damage to the temporal lobes of primates leads to the Klu-ver-Bucy syndrome, in which lesioned monkeys for example select and place in their mouths non-food as well as food items shown to them, and repeatedly fail to avoid noxious stimuli (Kluver and Bucy, 1939; Jones and Mishkin, 1972; Aggleton and Passingham, 1982; Baylis and Gaffan, 1991). Rats with lesions in the basolateral amygdala also display altered food selection, in that they ingest rel-atively novel foods, and do not learn to avoid normally ingesting a solution which has previously resulted in sickness. (The deficit in learned taste avoidance in rats may be due to damage to the insular taste cortex, which has projections through and to the amygdala – Dunn and Everitt, 1988). The basis for these alterations in food selection and in food-related learning are considered next (see also Rolls, 1992, 1994).

The monkeys with temporal lobe damage have a visual discrimi-nation deficit, in that they are impaired in learning to select one of two objects under which food is found, and thus fail to form correctly an association between the visual stimulus and reinforcement (Jones and Mishkin, 1972; Gaffan, 1992). Gaffan and Harrison (1987) and Gaffan et al. (1988) have shown that the tasks which are impaired by amygdala lesions in monkeys typically involve a cross-modal associ-ation from a previously neutral stimulus to a primary reinforcing stimulus (such as the taste of food), consistent with the hypothesis that the amygdala is involved in learning associations between stim-uli and primary reinforcers. Further evidence linking the amygdala to reinforcement mechanisms is that monkeys will work in order to obtain electrical stimulation of the amygdala, and that single neurons in the amygdala are activated by brain-stimulation reward of a num-ber of different sites (Rolls, 1975; Rolls et al., 1980).

The Kluver-Bucy syndrome is produced by lesions which damage the cortical areas in the anterior part of the temporal lobe and the underlying amygdala (Jones and Mishkin, 1972), or by lesions of the amygdala (Weiskrantz, 1956; Aggleton and Passingham, 1981; Gaffan, 1992), or of the temporal lobe neocortex (Akert et al., 1961). Lesions to part of the temporal lobe neocortex, damaging the infe-rior temporal visual cortex and extending into the cortex in the ven-tral bank of the superior temporal sulcus, produce visual aspects of the syndrome, seen for example as a tendency to select non-food as well as food items (Weiskrantz and Saunders, 1984). Anatomically, there are connections from the inferior temporal visual cortex and the orbitofrontal cortex to the amygdala, which in turn projects to the hypothalamus, thus providing a route for visual information to reach the hypothalamus (see Amaral et al., 1992). This evidence, together with the evidence that damage to the hypothalamus can disrupt feeding (see Winn et al., 1984; Clark et al., 1991; Le Magnen, 1992), thus indicates that there is a system which includes visual cortex in the temporal lobe, projections to the amygdala, and further connections to structures such as the lateral hypothalamus, which is involved in behavioral responses made on the basis of learned associations between visual stimuli and primary (unlearned) reinforcers such as the taste of food.

Analyses of neuronal responses in these different regions indicate that the inferior temporal visual cortex contains neurons that reflect the physical properties of visual stimuli but not their association with (taste) reward, and that the amygdala contains some visual neurons that reflect the taste reward association (Rolls, 1992); but that the region in primates which has neurons which mediate the very rapid learning of the association between the sight of a stimulus and its food reward value is in the orbitofrontal cortex, which is necessary for this rapid learning (Rolls, 1992, 1996). The ability to flexibly alter responses to stimuli based on their changing reinforcement associations is important in motivated behaviour (such as feeding) and in emotional behaviour, and it is this flexibility, it is suggested, that the orbitofrontal cortex, which develops greatly in primates, adds to a more basic capacity which the amygdala implements for stimulus-reinforcement learning.

Wilson and Rolls (see Rolls, 1992) extended the analysis of the responses of the amygdala neurons by showing that while they do respond to (some) stimuli associated with primary reinforcement, they do not respond if the reinforcement must be determined on the basis of a rule (such as that stimuli when novel are negatively reinforced, and when familiar are positively reinforced). This is consistent with the evidence that the amygdala is involved when reward must be determined, as normally occurs during feeding, by association of a stimulus with a primary reinforcer such as the taste of food, but is not involved when reinforcement must be determined in some other ways (see Gaffan, 1992; Rolls, 1992). In the same study, it was shown that these amygdala neurons which respond to food can also respond to some other stimuli while they are relatively novel. It is suggested that it is by this mechanism that when relatively novel stimuli are encountered, they are investigated, e.g., by being smelled and then placed in the mouth, to assess whether the new stimuli are foods (see Rolls, 1992).

Conclusion

Sensory-specific satiety, which occurs for the sight, taste and smell of food, is an important factor in determining food selection, especially during a meal. There is a long-term form of sensory-specific satiety which becomes evident when humans eat the same foods for long periods. The brain mechanisms which compute sensory-specific satiety are, in primates, largely in the orbitofrontal cortex. The primate orbitofrontal cortex is the brain region in which taste and olfactory signals combine to form the flavour of food. In the same brain region, visual and texture inputs combine with flavour signals, to form, by learned associations, representations of environmental stimuli which signify food, and are involved in food selection.

Acknowledgement

This research was supported by the Medical Research Council, Ref: PG8513790.

References

Aggleton, J.P. and Passingham, R.E. (1981) Syndrome produced by lesions of the amygdala in monkeys (Macaca mulatta), *Journal of Comparative Physiological Psychology*, 95: 961-977

Aggleton, J.P. and Passingham, R.E. (1982) An assessment of the reinforcing properties of foods after amygdaloid lesions in rhesus monkeys, *Journal of Comparative Physiological Psychology*, 96: 71-77

Akert, K., Gruesen, R.A., Woolsey, C.N. and Meyer, D.R. (1961) Kluver-Bucy syndrome in monkeys with neocortical ablations of temporal lobe, *Brain*, 84: 480-98

Amaral, D.G., Price, J.L., Pitkanen, A. and Carmichael, S.T. (1992) Anatomical organization of the primate amygdaloid complex, in J.P. Aggleton (ed.), *The Amygdala*, Wiley-Liss, New York, Ch.1: 1-66

Baylis, L.L. and Gaffan, D. (1991) Amygdalectomy and ventromedial prefrontal ablation produce similar deficits in food choice and in simple object discrimination learning for an unseen reward, *Experimental Brain Research*, 86: 617-22

Baylis, L.L. and Rolls, E.T. (1991) Responses of neurons in the primate taste cortex to glutamate, *Physiology and Behavior*, 49: 973-9

Butter, C.M., McDonald, J.A. and Snyder, D.R. (1969) Orality, preference behavior, and reinforcement value of non-food objects in monkeys with orbital frontal lesions, *Science*, 164: 1,306-7

Cabanac, M. (1971) Physiological role of pleasure, *Science*, 173: 1,103-7

Clark, J.M., Clark, A.J.M., Bartle, A. and Winn, P. (1991) The regulation of feeding and drinking in rats with lesions of the lateral hypothalamus made by N-methyl-D-aspartate, *Neuroscience*, 45: 631-40

Critchley, H.D. and Rolls, E.T. (1996a) Hunger and satiety modify the responses of olfactory and visual neurons in the primate orbitofrontal cortex, *Journal of Neurophysiology*, 75: 1,673-86

Critchley, H.D. and Rolls, E.T. (1996b) Responses of primate taste cortex neurons to the astringent tastant tannic acid, *Chemical Senses*, 21: 135-45

Dunn, L.T. and Everitt, B.J. (1988) Double dissociations of the effects of amygdala and insular cortex lesions on conditioned taste aversion, passive avoidance, and neophobia in the rat using the excitotoxin ibotenic acid, *Behavioural Neuroscience*, 102: 3-23

Gaffan, D. (1992) Amygdala and the memory of reward, in J.P. Aggleton (ed.), *The Amygdala*, Wiley-Liss, New York, Ch.18: 471-83

Gaffan, D., Gaffan, E.A., and Harrison S. (1989) Visual-visual associative learning and reward-association learning in monkeys: the role for the amygdala, *Journal of Neuroscience*, 9: 558-564

Gaffan, E.A., Gaffan, D. and Harrison, S. (1988) Disconnection of the amygdala from visual association cortex impairs visual reward-association learning in monkeys, *Journal of Neuroscience*, 8: 3,144-50

Gaffan, D. and Harrison, S. (1987) Amygdalectomy and disconnection in visual learning for auditory secondary reinforcement by monkeys, *Journal of Neuroscience*, 7: 2,285-92

Jones, B. and Mishkin, M. (1972) Limbic lesions and the problem of stimulus-reinforcement associations, *Experimental Neurology*, 36: 362-77

Kluver, H. and Bucy, P.C. (1939) Preliminary analysis of functions of the temporal lobes in monkeys, *Archives of Neurological Psychiatry*, 42: 979-1000

Le Magnen, J. (1992) *Neurobiology of Feeding and Nutrition*, Academic Press, San Diego

Mora, F., Rolls, E.T. and Burton, M.J. (1976) Modulation during learning of the responses of neurons in the hypothalamus to the sight of food, *Experimental Neurology*, 53: 508-19

Rolls, B.J. and Hetherington, M. (1989) The role of variety in eating and body weight regulation, in R. Shepherd (ed.), *Handbook of the Psychophysiology of Human Eating*, Wiley, Chichester, 57-84

Rolls, B.J., Rolls, E.T., Rowe, E.A. and Sweeney, K. (1981) Sensory specific satiety in man, *Physiology and Behaviour*, 27: 137-42

Rolls, B.J., Rowe, E.A. and Rolls, E.T. (1982) How sensory properties of foods affect human feeding behavior, *Physiology and Behavior*, 29: 409-17

Rolls, B.J., Van Duijenvoorde, P.M. and Rowe, E.A. (1983) Variety in the diet enhances intake in a meal and contributes to the development of obesity in the rat, *Physiology and Behavior*, 31: 21-7

Rolls, B.J., Van Duijenvoorde, P.M. and Rolls, E.T. (1984) Pleasantness changes and food intake in a varied four course meal, *Appetite*, 5: 337-48

Rolls, E.T. (1975) *The Brain and Reward*, Pergamon, Oxford

Rolls, E.T. (1989) Information processing in the taste system of primates, *Journal of Experimental Biology*, 146, 141-64

Rolls, E.T. (1992) Neurophysiology and functions of the primate amygdala, in J.P. Aggleton (ed.), *The Amygdala*, Wiley-Liss, New York, 143-65

Rolls, E.T. (1993) Neurophysiology of feeding in primates, in D.A. Booth (ed.), *Neurophysiology of Ingestion*, Pergamon, Oxford, 137-69

Rolls, E.T. (1994) Neural processing related to feeding in primates, in C.R. Legg and D.A. Booth (eds.), *Appetite: Neural and Behavioural Bases*, Oxford University Press, 11-53

Rolls, E.T. (1995) Central taste anatomy and physiology, in R.L. Doty (ed.), *Handbook of Olfaction and Gustation*, Dekker, New York, 549-573

Rolls, E.T. (1996) The orbitofrontal cortex, *Philosophical Transactions of the Royal Society*, 351: 1433-44

Rolls, E.T. and Baylis, L.L. (1994) Gustatory, olfactory and visual convergence within the primate orbitofrontal cortex, *Journal of Neuroscience*, 14: 5437-52

Rolls, E.T., Burton, M.J. and Mora, F. (1980) Neurophysiological analysis of brain-stimulation reward in the monkey, *Brain Research*, 194: 339-57

Rolls, E.T. and de Waal, A.W.L. (1985) Long-term sensory-specific satiety: evidence from an Ethiopian refugee camp, *Physiology and Behavior*, 34: 1017-20

Rolls, E.T., Rolls, B.J. and Rowe, E.A. (1983) Sensory-specific and motivation-specific satiety for the sight and taste of food and water in man, *Physiology and Behavior*, 30: 185-92

Rolls, E.T. and Rolls, J.H. (1997) Olfactory and taste sensory-specific satiety in humans, *Physiology and Behavior*, 61: 461-473

Rolls, E.T., Sienkiewicz, Z.J., and Yaxley, S. (1989) Hunger modulates the responses to gustatory stimuli of single neurons in the caudolateral orbitofrontal cortex of the macaque monkey, *European Journal of Neuroscience*, 1: 53-60

Rolls, E.T. and Treves, A. (1997) *Neural Networks and Brain Function*, Oxford University Press

Takagi, S.F. (1991) Olfactory frontal cortex and multiple olfactory processing in primates, in A. Peters and E.G. Jones (eds.), *Cerebral Cortex* 9, Plenum Press, New York, 133-52

Thorpe, S.J., Rolls, E.T. and Maddison, S. (1983) Neuronal activity in the orbitofrontal cortex of the behaving monkey, *Experimental Brain Research*, 49: 93-115

Weiskrantz, L. (1956) Behavioral changes associated with ablation of the amygdaloid complex in monkeys, *Journal of Comparative Physiological Psychology*, 49: 381-91

Weiskrantz, L. and Saunders, R.C. (1984) Impairments of visual object transforms in monkeys, *Brain*, 107: 1033-72

Wilson, F.A.W. and Rolls, E.T. (1990) Neuronal responses related to reinforcement in the primate basal forebrain, *Brain Research*, 502: 213-31

Winn, P., Tarbuck, A. and Dunnett, S.B. (1984) Ibotenic acid lesions of the lateral hypothalamus: comparison with electrolytic lesion syndrome, *Neuroscience*, 12: 225-40

5. GOOD TASTE AND BAD TASTE
PREFERENCES AND AVERSIONS AS BIOLOGICAL PRINCIPLES

Wulf Schiefenhövel

Disgust is an emotion which regulates perceptions and behaviours in a wide range of situations. Many, but not all of them, have to do with food, eating and drinking. In this contribution I propose the hypothesis that disgust is also instrumental in the nutritional niches which human populations occupy. In this respect disgust is a powerful principle leading to cultural diversity. While the first part of the chapter discusses the neurobiology of the disgust emotion, I go on to consider anthropological consequences and to suggest a hypothesis in regard to ecological niches.

External Signs of Disgust

Disgust is one of the six basic emotions, the universality of which is now acknowledged even by hard-core behavioural psychologists. The facial expression of disgust is mainly brought about by the contraction of the *Musculus levator labii superioris*. Hjortsjö (1970) was the first to identify clearly, through careful anatomical and functional analysis, the smallest independent units of muscle actions in the face. He numbered these neuromuscular units. Ekman and Friesen later adopted this method and turned it into the now much used Facial Action Coding System (F.A.C.S.) (Ekman and Friesen, 1978). The *M. levator labii superioris* pulls, according to the vector of its action, the middle part of the upper lip upwards. This movement causes the

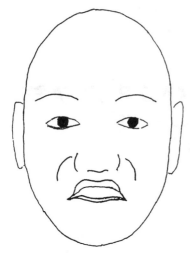

Figure 5.1 Action unit 10, the facial expression of disgust
(*Source*: adapted from Hjortsjö, 1970)

nasolabial furrow to change its normal appearance (a more or less straight line obliquely running down from the corner of the nose to the corner of the mouth) to become an inverted U (Figure 5.1). In strong signs of disgust the mouth is often opened through a drop of the lower jaw and the tongue is stuck out (Figure 5.2).

Common stimuli answered by the disgust face are rotten substances with a putrid smell, body wastes, especially faeces, and slimy fluids. Apart from these – I argue – natural releasers, disgust is triggered by a whole lot of psychological and social situations as well as mental states. Notwithstanding these many shades of meaning the expression of disgust can have, it is possible to trace them back to a biopsychological origin. The full blown disgust face matches very well the facial expression connected to vomiting. The mouth is opened and the tongue is stuck out to facilitate the discharge of the contents of stomach and, in some cases, duodenum. This is the facial expression that Rozin et al. in the next chapter describe as the 'gape'.

We are dealing here with one of the interesting ritualisations (in the ethological sense) of a reflex-type action within the body for the sake of non-verbal communication. In the physiological domain, i.e., that connected to the primary releasers, rotten and repulsive substances, as described above, the neurobiology of the disgust-emotion shifted to become a purely social signal. This has, in the process of hominisation, happened with other facial action units as well (see Schiefenhövel et al., 1994).

Nature is parsimonious. Once a neuromuscular pathway was established (in this case to facilitate the act of vomiting),

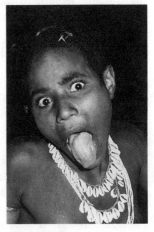

Figure 5.2 Eipo woman signalling strong rejection with full disgust face – a ritualised act of vomiting (*Photograph*: W. Schiefenhövel)

this pathway could be used for non-physiological purposes as well. From this perspective, the semantic message of the social disgust face becomes quite obvious: if I activate action unit ten, open the mouth and stick out the tongue, my interaction partner will intuitively understand that this is a very strong sign of rejection. I react, with the social disgust face, to my interaction partner as if he or she were one of the rotten, aversive substances which physiologically bring about the disgust reaction.

Figure 5.3 Variation in heart rate and skin temperature in an experimental situation in which the expression of six emotions was built up through instructions to move certain facial muscles. The other emotions led to an increase in heart frequency.

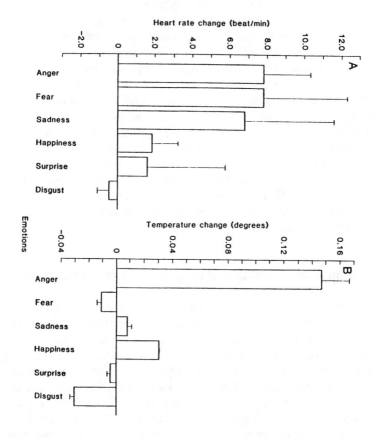

Note: Disgust, in contrast to all other emotions, led to a decrease in heart frequency (*Source:* adapted from Ekman et al., 1983)

This connection between the biological and the psychosocial domain is illustrated well by an experiment which was carried out by Ekman et al. (1983). Actors were equipped with a number of electrodes, measuring heart frequency, skin temperature, skin conductance, etc. One of the team of experts for facial expression then instructed these test volunteers to move certain parts of their face in specific directions. In this very technical way the expressions typical for the six basic emotions were produced, without any foregoing corresponding emotion, as the actors were not asked to make an angry, happy, disgusted or such face. One outcome of this experiment (Figure 5.3) was that there are indeed specific emotional states connected to specific psychophysiological parameters. Another important insight from this study is that it is possible 'artificially', by shaping certain facial movements, to create the corresponding emotions from outside to inside.

In the discussion of our topic here, another result of this study is the most interesting. Five of the six emotions produced a more or less marked increase in heart frequency. Only disgust showed a decrease. From a neuroanatomical, physiological perspective this outcome (overlooked by the original authors) can easily be explained. If the disgust face is, as is its ritualisation, causally connected to the act of vomiting, then the lowering of the heart frequency does not come as a surprise. The actual act of retching and vomiting is brought about by *Nervus glossopharyngeus* and *Nervus vagus*. The latter has a marked decreasing influence on the heart frequency. The experiment shows, thereby, that the interpretation of the disgust face as a ritualised act of vomiting is valid.

Having established a causal link between the social disgust face and the act of vomiting, it is now time to look at the internal physiological regulation of the disgust reaction.

The Internal Regulation of Disgust, Nausea and Emesis

As can be seen from the model of the brain centres (Figure 5.4), pathways and transmitter mechanisms known today to be involved in the regulation of the act of vomiting are part of a complex cybernetical system which most likely has many more single elements, plus feed forward and feed back loops, than we know of at the present time. A precursor of emesis (the act of vomiting) is nausea, the not very well defined but, strongly unpleasant feeling that something is wrong in one's inside. In the model above the 'chemoceptive triggerzone', also known as the *area postrema*, is an extremely interesting part of the brain. It is here that, in contrast to all other locations, the blood-brain-barrier is non-existent.

Figure 5.4 Central nervous system pathways involved in vomiting

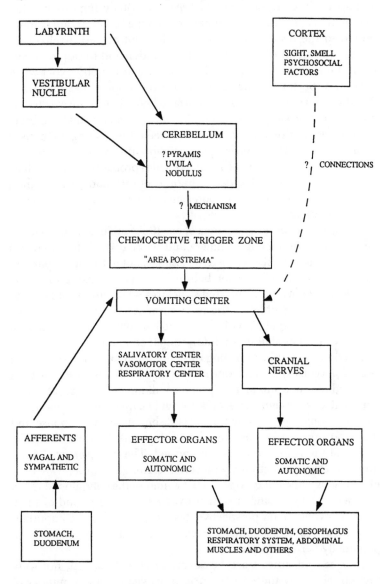

(*Source*: adapted from Wang & Chinn, 1956)

Thus, this special location functions to allow toxins and other harmful substances carried by the blood stream to reach the cells of the *area postrema* unfiltered. If this were to happen in the other parts of the brain, damage would ensue. But here, in the confined and specially equipped *area postrema*, the vitally important information that something wrong has entered the blood stream is transmitted to the brain and thereby to the centres and mechanisms which are able to react to this toxin condition and to stop or alleviate it. One of these measures is to vomit and thereby expel whatever may be left of the toxin inside the upper intestinal tract. Another, perhaps the most important behavioural answer to the message that toxins are reaching the *area postrema* is that the brain establishes a direct connection between the feeling of nausea induced in the *area postrema* plus neighbouring structures and the memory of the food last consumed. Smell is probably the most effective single factor to bring bad memories of this kind back: animals and humans will not eat this food again or will at least be very careful of it in future.

In a classic experiment Garcia et al. (1968) subjected rats to invisible X-rays. The feeling of illness and nausea which followed this experimental treatment caused the animals not to touch the particular food which they had eaten before the ill-feeling had started. The *area postrema* plus the connected structures which are most likely to have been responsible for the reaction of the animals are decisive elements in the regulation of aversion to harmful substances, most of which were, in evolutionary times, contained in food.

In contrast to other learning or conditioning mechanisms in the central nervous system the one represented by the *area postrema* does not need repeated stimuli to trigger a conditioned response. One bad experience is enough. A second unusual characteristic is that there can be a long time between the establishment of the response and the exposure to a second stimulus of the same nature without the power of the response being diminished. The *area postrema*, therefore, represents an extremely powerful learning response, with a single stimulus sufficient to trigger a behaviour of the conditioned reflex type which stays change-resistant over a very long period of time. From an evolutionary perspective this mechanism has the important function of protecting animals, including humans, from the intake of potentially harmful foods.

Nausea and emesis are however, as already stated, not only brought about by the *area postrema*. In its vicinity are a number of neuronal structures (Figure 5.5) which receive information particularly from the walls of the stomach and the duodenum. This whole region, situated on the floor of the fourth ventricle, consists of various pathways which transmit the results of primary data processing in this region to other parts of the brain.

Figure 5.5 Brain structures around the *area postrema*

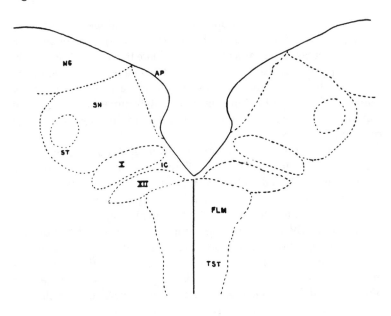

(*Source:* adapted from Morest, 1960)

As shown in Figure 5.4 hitherto more or less unknown neuronal connections exist between the cortex (and other parts of the brain) feeding memories, emotional qualities and moods into the complex cybernetic system dealing with nausea, emesis and, at the other end of the spectrum, pleasure from the intake of food and drink. As taste is, in its physiological quality, the outcome of an interplay between the taste buds in the tongue and the fine-grained olfactory information processed by the very ancient mammalian system to perceive smell, we must assume that another complex network of pathways is connected to the overall system regulating our evaluation of 'good' foods and 'bad' foods.

The *Nervus olfactorius,* an extremely simple nerve structurally, but with regard to its power of transmitting and processing the most detailed smell signals, an extraordinarily efficient one, projects its fibres directly into the limbic system. This is also one of the most ancient structures of the brain, developed in the course of evolution especially as a memory device. We humans, too, base many of our actions on affective evaluations which receive input from memories and especially their emotional qualities. Schleidt (1992) has shown how important olfactory engrammes of foods are for our subjective feeling of wellbeing.

Anthropological Consequences

It has become evident, I hope, that we are equipped with a very complex system for evaluating the wide range of specific qualities in foods. Whereas some parts of the system, like the *area postrema* mechanism, are more or less 'hard-wired' and have fixed biological mechanisms, other parts are very susceptible to various inputs during ontogeny. They are the entry ports for environmental, i.e., cultural stimuli, which then create the preferences and the aversions typical of human cultures.

The emotion of disgust is, especially during childhood, very 'contagious' i.e., easy to tap. Children will show the disgust face when one in the group has tried an unknown food and reacts (as usually happens to the despair of their parents) with the typical facial signs of aversion. The other children, without having had any material access to the food, will react with the same facial signs and stubbornly decline to eat this particular food, no matter how sweet the seductions that the adults attempt to employ. It is very likely that this contagiousness is not restricted to the facial expression of disgust, i.e., the outside signal, but that it is also able to elicit the psycho-physiological actions of the nausea-emesis reaction, the inside mechanism.

In children this may lead to being very conservative about the integration of new foods into the diet. In a functional view this can be seen as a possible biological protection mechanism and, at the same time, as one of the mechanisms constituting ethnicity, which is strongly rooted in preferences and aversions of taste.

In adults too, the disgust reaction seems to be triggered easily. Members of one ethnic group will often react with a disgust face and ritualised vomiting movements when speaking about other ethnic groups. This reaction is not limited to foods, but extended to a wide range of other socio-cultural markers, particularly ones which are subject to moral evaluation. The powerful biological disgust 'motor' can drive various wheels. The process of enculturation, which takes place during childhood and is somewhat reduced during later life, narrows down the wide spectrum of possible foods to the pattern typical for the specific culture.

Food customs of other cultures are very often evaluated on the crude basis of the disgust mechanism. The French tradition of eating horsemeat elicits this kind of response in many Germans and the same is true for the relationship between other ethnic groups on our planet. Chinese eating dogs and 'rotten eggs', Maasai drinking blood, and Europeans eating 'rotten milk' (cheese), are examples which could be continued in a very long list. One outcome of this biocultural mechanism for food preferences and aversions is that ethnic groups are niching themselves into given ecological environments.

The Disgust Reaction and Ecological Niches

Take the Trobriand islanders for example. The people of the northern villages on the main rather densely populated island of Kiriwina with its many inland settlements are known to be very efficient at catching sharks *(kwau)* by using special hooks plus techniques to attract the fish. In other areas of Melanesia, e.g., New Ireland, a different, more spectacular method is used, which involves causing the shark to come out of the water close to the out-rigger canoe so that the loop of a trap can be placed, by bare hands, over their heads.

On the other hand, the villagers of Tauwema on the small island of Kaileuna, and their neighbours, who have easy access to a rich variety of coral fish plus tuna and similar species from deeper waters, do not catch shark with hooks and consider their meat inferior or outright disgusting. When the crew of a boat has killed a shark, usually by hitting the fish with a paddle, the meat is not usually consumed by them. The villagers say that it has an aversive smell and taste. Indeed, sharks do not have the 'modern' renal system of other vertebrates and utilise part of the urea in their blood to build up osmotic pressure to equal that of the seawater. Shark meat, therefore, has a little of the smell and taste of this urea. This fact constitutes one of the criteria on which the non-sharkeaters reject this valuable source of protein, whereas the shark eaters are not bothered by it or even have a preference for this kind of meat. Other criteria are also involved: larger shark species are potentially dangerous for humans, and members of the shark family, therefore, evoke generally negative feelings.

For the marine ecology around the Trobriand Islands this differentiation of resource utilisation is most likely to have marked effects. Sharks are only caught for consumption in a confined area. This may have a protective effect on the marine fauna of which certain species are diminished regionally but can multiply elsewhere. Yet, seen from a systemic biological perspective, these effects are probably quite small for the ecology around the Trobriand Islands. In other areas of the world, however, such effects may be of important dimensions.

Conclusion

For the Trobrianders, eating versus not eating shark is important on a symbolic and human ethological level. Through such a mix of physiologically and socially triggered disgust, cultural markers are established. This principle of building ethnicity through the described biopsychological mechanism is widespread, probably universal in the cultures of our planet. In this way a neuromuscular pathway, which originally evolved for physiological benefit, becomes the social disgust face, signalling disgust to others as well as self. It is, furthermore, argued in this chapter that the disgust expressed about the eating preferences of other groups is frequently used as an ethnic marker and thereby fosters exploitation of different ecological niches.

References

Ekman, P. and Friesen, W. (1978) *Facial Action Coding System*, Consulting Psychologists Press, Palo Alto

Ekman, P., Levenson, R.W., Friesen, W. (1983) Autonomic nervous system activity distinguishes among emotions, *Science* 221: 1,208-10

Garcia J., McGowan, B.K., Ervin, F.R. und Koelling, R.A. (1968) Cues: their relative effectiveness as a function of the reinforcer, *Science*, 160: 794-5

Hjortsjö, C.H. (1970) Man's Face and Mimic, *Language*, Studentlitteratur, Lund

Morest, D.K. (1960) A study of the structure of the *area postrema* with Golgi methods, *American Journal of Anatomy*, 107: 291-303

Schiefenhövel, W., Vogel, Ch., Vollmer, G. & Opolka U. (eds.) (1994) Zwischen Natur und Kultur, *Der Mensch und seine Beziehungen*, Trias, Stuttgart

Schleidt, M. (1992) The semiotic relevance of human olfaction: A biological approach, in S. van Troller and G.H. Dodd (eds.), *Fragance: The Psychology and Biology of Perfume*, Elsevier, London, 37-50

Wang, S.C. and Chinn H.I. (1956) Experimental motion sickness in dogs: Importance of labyrinth and vestibular cerebellum, *American Journal of Physiology*, 185: 617-23

6. DISGUST
PREADAPTATION AND THE CULTURAL EVOLUTION OF A FOOD-BASED EMOTION

Paul Rozin, Jonathan Haidt, Clark McCauley and *Sumio Imada*

There has been a tendency in recent years to try to account for human behaviour in any domain as either highly constrained by biology or entirely socially constructed. In this chapter, we will make an effort to establish what we think is a reasonable middle ground. We describe how a food-rejection system, strongly rooted in mammalian biology, has been elaborated and transformed to become a distinctively human emotion. The biological roots of the transformed emotion are still apparent in its facial expressions, its characteristic behaviour (withdrawal), and its physiological correlate (nausea), but the meaning and elicitors of the emotion are totally transformed by culture. In brief, a mammalian mechanism for rejecting distasteful and noxious foods, a system which protects the body from harm, is transformed into a uniquely human mechanism for internalising cultural rules and, ultimately, we suggest, the protection of the human soul.

We identify the process through which these changes occur as an instance of preadaptation (a system/property evolved to perform one function is subsequently shared or coopted for another function). Preadaptation was originally advanced as a mechanism of biological evolution (Bock, 1959; Mayr, 1961; Rozin, 1976), but we apply it here to the cultural evolution of disgust. The cultural-historical trajectory of the emotion of disgust illustrates how a food-specific system forms a base, a biological and cultural metaphor, for a much larger domain of preadaptation.

This kind of trajectory should be no surprise, because our complex sociocultural world must grow out of fundamental and largely innate biological processes, such as eating, sex, and sleeping. In the domain of eating, in particular, basic processes attain a high level of abstraction and a wide range of generality. The 'smile' to palatable tastes (Steiner, 1979; Chiva, 1985) becomes invoked as an interaction facilitator, the vocabulary of taste (sweet, bitter and sour) become metaphors to describe a wide range of experiences (Lakoff and Johnson, 1980), and the distaste gape (drop of lower jaw), becomes a general expression of rejection from the self.

Given the wide range of applications of the word 'disgust' or its rough synonyms in other languages, it may not be obvious that this emotion is, at its core, about food. However, the name itself, disgust (and similar names in some other languages) means bad taste, the facial expression is similar to the expression made by animals and human infants that serves to expel food from the mouth, and the physiological manifestation of disgust – nausea – is uniquely effective in discouraging ingestion.

Origins of Disgust in Distaste

We believe that disgust originates in the gape response, seen in a variety of animals (Grill and Norgren, 1977) and newborn human infants (Steiner, 1979; Rosenstein and Oster, 1988) in response to innately distasteful substances. The bitter taste is probably the prototype for eliciting this distaste response. This piece of mammalian biology may, itself, qualify as an emotion according to some definitions commonly used. It involves a specific set of functional behaviours: withdrawal or ridding the body of an undesirable substance. There are distinctive functional facial (and bodily) movements, with expressive qualities and a likely communicative functions. There is reason to believe that, as with adult humans, these expressions are associated with the experience of nausea (see Rozin and Fallon, 1987; Rozin et al., 1993, for more details). It also seems reasonable also to presume that the feeling of revulsion experienced by humans may have a counterpart in other mammals showing the distaste response. We will call the distaste response a proto-emotion.

Elaboration of Food Rejection Systems in Humans

Our analysis of the basis of food rejection in adults (Fallon & Rozin, 1983) suggests that there are three kinds of motive leading to rejection of potential foods by humans. One is distaste, that is, undesirable sensory properties (taste, smell, visual) of a substance. A second is anticipated consequences, what we have learned are the negative effects of eating certain substances. A third is conceptual, what we know about the nature or origin of substances.

These three motivations develop gradually, with only the distaste system present at birth. We believe that as other motives come in, the basis for food rejection becomes elaborated in development (Fallon, Rozin & Pliner, 1984; Rozin, Fallon & Augustoni-Ziskind, 1986). In the first years of life, children learn that some substances are not good for them. They either directly experience discomfort upon eating these substances or they learn from others to expect such discomfort. We identify these substances, rejected on account of anticipated negative consequences, as dangers (as opposed to distastes).

With growing sophistication and awareness, children learn that certain things are not to be eaten because they are not food (a conceptual distinction), even though they may cause no harm. We call such items inappropriate substances; the category includes earth, paper and tree bark.

Finally, in the age range of perhaps four to eight years in American culture, the more sophisticated form of conceptual rejection emerges that we call disgust. Disgusting foods are rejected principally because of conceptual reasons – their nature or origin. However, they are also believed to taste bad, and they are often thought to be harmful. So disgust can invoke all three motivations, at least in many cases (see Rozin, Fallon & Augustoni-Ziskind, 1986 for details on the development of disgust in children). Disgust is arguably the strongest form of food rejection.

Disgust, as we define it, is distinctively different from the other categories of food rejection (Table 6.1). Disgust shares with distaste a facial expression and perhaps the nausea response, but the basis of disgust is not primarily sensory. Thus, although we see disgust as originating in distaste, we see disgust as already qualitatively different from distaste for children in the early school years. Lima beans may be distasteful (to some), but no one thinks they are offensive; if they tasted different, or were swallowed whole with a tasty coating, they would be acceptable. Not so for worms, because it is not their taste that ultimately offends us, but their 'wormness'. The conceptual rejection characteristic of disgust is a notable cognitive achievement; disgust depends on the conception of an essence (wormness) that exists independent of any sensory qualities.

Core Disgust

We call the disgust response, as we have described it in American adults, core disgust (Rozin and Fallon, 1987; Rozin et al., 1993). Our working definition of core disgust derives from the definition provided by Angyal (1941) in his seminal paper on disgust. It is: 'Revulsion at the prospect of (oral) incorporation of an offensive object. The offensive objects are contaminants; that is, if they even briefly contact an acceptable food, they tend to render that food unacceptable' (Rozin and Fallon, 1987: 23).

There are three critical parts of this definition. The first part, oral incorporation, refers directly to eating and reflects the fact that eating is the principal way in which we materially incorporate the outside world into the self. This is, not surprisingly, an act that is laden with affect. We trace the intimacy of this act to the material invasion of the self that is involved in eating, and in particular, to the widespread traditional belief that one takes on the properties of what one eats – 'you are what you eat' (Rozin and Fallon, 1987). We have shown that there is an implicit belief of this sort even in educated American adults (Nemeroff and Rozin, 1989).

A second critical part of the definition is the idea of an offensive substance. It should be clear from the 'you are what you eat' principle that if one eats something offensive, one becomes offensive. Hence the reluctance to consume offensive substances. But what makes something offensive? Angyal (1941) proposed that animal waste products are the central elicitors of disgust and suggested that faeces are the universal disgust substance. Unlike bitter aversion, the aversion to faeces seems to be acquired (Petó, 1936; Rozin, Hammer, Oster, Horowitz and Marmara, 1986).

We have expanded Angyal's proposal to suggest that the central domain of disgust elicitors includes all animals and their products when considered as food (Rozin and Fallon, 1987). Almost all food-related disgust elicitors for Americans are animals or animal products: insects, reptiles, cats, dogs, mice, rats, monkeys, any kind of rotten flesh, and most animal products except cow's milk and chicken eggs. Of course, in most cultures, some animals or animal products, almost always a very small minority of the total types available, become desirable foods. But these exceptions, which for Americans include only a few parts or products of a few animal species, only underline the rule against eating animals. In the light of the 'you are what you eat' principle, one might say that humans feel threatened that they might become too 'animal-like', as a result of consuming other animals or their products.

The third part of the definition is contamination. Our analysis suggests that contamination is a manifestation of the law of contagion originally described by the anthropologists Tylor (1871), Frazer (1890/1959) and Mauss (1902/1962; see Rozin and Neneraffm 1990, for a review). This law was described originally as a belief typical of traditional societies: once two entities make physical contact, essential properties of each pass permanently between them ('once in contact, always in contact'). We have shown that the law of contagion appears even in the behaviour of American adults (Rozin, Millman and Nemeroff, 1986). That is, Americans are inclined to reject foods that have contacted a disgusting entity, such as a worm, cockroach or body waste product. The deep motivation in these rejections seems not to be fear of microbial infection, because the rejection is not substantially weakened if the disgusting contaminating agent is sterilized. The intuition here, even for educated Westerners, is that when a cockroach touches their mashed potatoes, even briefly with no visible residue, the potatoes have been 'cockroached' and take on some cockroach properties.

The coupling of the 'you are what you eat' principle with the law of contagion greatly enlarges the domain of contamination (Rozin, 1990). Thus, when an undesirable person prepares a food, that food is contaminated; subsequent ingestion of that food passes the offensive properties on to the consumer by the 'you are what you eat' principle. Hence, a chain of indirect human influences may be brought to bear on the process of eating, as happens most saliently in Hindu Indian culture (Marriott, 1968; Appadurai, 1981) and among the Hua of Papua New Guinea (Meigs, 1984).

It is our belief, indicated in the designation 'core disgust', that revulsion to animals and body products in the context of food is the primary and ontogenetically earliest expression of disgust. The core disgust system is constructed from the preadapted distaste food rejection system. The modification of this system involves a change in meaning and elicitors. Core disgust shares some of the properties of distaste, including the facial expression, behavioural withdrawal and nausea, but disgust differs qualitatively from distaste in both the presence of contamination and the sense of conceptually based offensiveness. The principal elicitors of core disgust are animals and animal products in a food context (Table 6.1).

Animal Nature Disgust

We have asked American adult subjects to list some examples of things that they consider disgusting, and Japanese adults to do the same with respect to the closest Japanese synonym to disgust that we can find (*ken'o*). In both cultures, only about one-quarter of the responses can be classified as core disgust (Haidt, Rozin, McCauley and Imada, 1997). Many of the remaining instances can be classified into one of the following four domains:

1. poor hygiene;
2. inappropriate sexual activities (e.g., between people of very different ages, or between people and animals);
3. body envelope violations (gore);
4. contact with death.

We have constructed a scale to measure individual differences in disgust sensitivity (Haidt, McCauley and Rozin, 1994). This scale includes instances that represent each of the seven domains of disgust we have mentioned (animals, food, body products, poor hygiene, sex, gore and death) and some items tapping contagion sensitivity as well. We find wide variations in disgust sensitivity in both American and Japanese respondents, with a high degree of similarity in the range of scores and item responses in Japan and the United States (Imada, Haidt, McCauley and Rozin, n.d.).

Wronska (1990) has independently constructed a disgust scale in Poland, and her scale is remarkably similar to our own in terms of the domains of disgust elicitors represented. Although her particular items were often quite different from ours in ways that reflect the rural environment of Poland (e.g., smell of a manure pit), her items could easily be recognised as representing five of our domains of elicitors: food, animals, body products, sex, and hygiene.

In examining our seven domains of disgust elicitors, we note that a common feature is that each domain refers to something physical that humans share with animals: basic body functions such as eating and sex, body care (with lack of cleanliness associated with animals), body excretions such as faeces and mucous, a body envelope that can be cut or ripped to reveal mushy insides (gore), and a body destined for death and putrefaction. This common feature is consistent with a suggestion made by Rozin and Fallon (1987) that one aspect of disgusting substances is that they are reminders of our animal nature.

There is abundant evidence from ethnographies that humans see themselves as qualitatively different from, and superior to, 'animals' (e.g., Leach, 1964; Tambiah, 1969). Reminders of our animal nature are unpleasant, and are to be rejected from the mind just as offensive foods are rejected from the mouth. Hence, we propose that, in both individual development and in cultural evolution, the already developed (preadapted) core disgust rejection system is expanded to include animal nature reminders (Rozin, Haidt and McCauley, 1993). In our account, animal origin disgust represents a second evolution of the emotion of disgust (Table 6.1).

Table 6.1 Proposed Pathway of Expansion of Disgust and Disgust Elicitors

			Disgust stage		
	Distaste	Core	Animal nature	Interpersonal contamination	Moral
Function	Protect body	Protect body and soul	Protect body and soul	Protect body, soul, and social order	Protect social order
Eliciters	Bad tastes	Food/eating, body products, animals	Sex, death, hygiene, envelope violations	Direct and indirect contact with strangers or undesirables	Certain moral offences

Death and Disgust

Examination of the relationships between each of the thirty-two questions on the disgust scale and the total score on the test reveals that some of the best predictors of the total score are individual items that deal with death, such as being disgusted by touching a corpse or picking up a dead pet cat (Haidt, McCauley and Rozin, 1994). The salience of death sensitivity fits well with the fact that the quintessential stimulus feature prompting disgust is the smell of decay. Furthermore, *miasma*, the ancient Greek concept akin to our concept of pollution, was prototypically engaged by contact with death (Parker, 1983). A critical role for death in disgust is further supported by the centrality of mortality in human psychological functioning, as argued by Ernest Becker in *The Denial of Death* (1973). Becker, taking a psychodynamic approach, argues that the main function of our defence mechanisms is to suppress the thought or realisation of our own mortality. He holds that it is our mortality, rather than our sexual or aggressive impulses, that represents the fundamental human dilemma. In this perspective (see Rozin, Haidt and McCauley, 1993 for more details), death becomes *hweder* the animal property that is most threatening to humans. Thus, a second account of animal nature disgust gives a central place to denial of death, with disgust serving to keep such thoughts out of the mind.

Although we are suggesting that disgust is an emotion that functions to keep away intimations of our mortality, we do not want to

go so far as to suggest that all experiences involving disgust are likewise avoided. Toy stores sell disgusting toys – imitation mucus, crea-
tures that vomit – to school-aged boys. Film makers sell horror films
and slasher films that probably elicit a good deal of disgust from
their mostly adolescent audiences. Funerals and other rituals such as
circumcision probably elicit disgust in at least some adult participants. Public interest in and discussion of crimes of violence is often
high, as in the case of Jeffrey Dahmer who killed, dismembered, and
ate at least ten people. Evidently, disgusting experiences are not
always avoided.

The examples just cited all involve experience of disgust in a social
situation: the toys, the films, the rituals and the news are used in interactions with others. It seems possible that sharing and comparing disgust reactions can be the source of a social bond or attraction that
distinguishes the ingroup from outgroups. In this way shared disgust
can be a celebration of the barrier between animal and human even
as this barrier keeps out thoughts of our animal origins. The chapter
by Schiefenhövel in this volume points in a similar direction.

Interpersonal Disgust

Some disgust elicitors do not fit within the category of animal nature
reminders. These include certain moral violations and a wide range
of direct and indirect physical contacts with other people (Table 6.1).
We consider these two final domains of elicitors in this and the next
section. We have no suggestion as to an ordering of these two
domains, either in individual development or in cultural evolution.

Although it is not commonly suggested by subjects spontaneously
offering examples of disgust, contact with undesirable persons is
reliably considered both disgusting and contaminating (Haidt,
McCauley and Rozin, 1994). In a questionnaire study of American
adults, for instance, Rozin, Markwith and McCauley (1994) asked
how much respondents would like to use each of three objects previously used by a target person: a sweater (laundered), a hotel bed
(with clean linen), and a used car. The target person (previous user)
was described as, in different instances, a healthy stranger, a person
with tuberculosis (illness), a person with an amputated leg (misfortune) and a person who was a healthy convicted murderer (moral
taint). A substantial minority of subjects rated the item used by the
healthy stranger as considerably less attractive than a new item.
Much more negative ratings were found for used objects when the
previous user had experienced misfortune or had a disease or moral

taint. These more negative responses were characteristic of almost all subjects (even though the sweater was laundered, and the bed linen changed). The results clearly indicate a strong negativity (we read this as disgust) to any physical contact, even indirect, with an undesirable person.

Of course, the healthy stranger does not have any obvious undesirable properties. Further analysis indicates that elimination of any presumed negative properties of a stranger (e.g., by specifying that the person is a priest or is physically attractive) has little effect on those people who find stranger contact aversive/disgusting (McCauley, Rozin, and Markwith, n.d.). It seems that even indirect contact with unknown others can elicit disgust for many Americans. This can be interpreted as a self-protecting impulse, an aversion/disgust aimed at distancing the self from others, particularly different or strange others. Again we note that Schiefenhövel's paper in this volume comes independently to the view that disgust in humans serves as an ethnic or outgroup marker.

If we consider disgust as an expression of revulsion and a distancing of the self from a disgust elicitor, then it becomes an emotion much involved in both individuation and, by its absence, an expression of solidarity. This leads us to predict major differences in the interpersonal aspects of disgust in cultures that vary in interpersonal attitudes. Markus and Kitayama (1991) have recently summarised evidence suggesting a major difference between Japanese and Americans on this dimension, with Japanese characterised as having an interdependent self, in contrast to an American independent self. We do not yet know enough about the boundaries that define interdependence (other members of the family, friends, members of the local community, or all Japanese), but we would expect that the domain of interpersonal disgust in Japan might be quite different from that in the United States.

Furthermore, interpersonal deference and harmonious relationships have particular value in Japan. Hence, any violation of social interaction rules might be considered more serious and even disgusting in Japan. There is some support for this possibility in the spontaneous examples of *ken'o* offered by Japanese subjects (Haidt, Rozin, McCauley and Imada, 1994). These examples include instances of failure in the management of everyday social interactions, such as 'when I was betrayed by a person I trusted' or 'when others around me took no notice of me' (Imada, Yamada and Haidt, 1993).

In Hindu India, the domain of interpersonal disgust may take on a yet more important and distinctive form. In general, Hindu Indians seem more concerned about interpersonal than 'animal' pollution. That is, the focus of disgust in Hindu India may be more on interpersonal and moral elicitors than on the animal nature and core disgust categories. This probably results from the high respect in which many animals are held, and to beliefs about reincarnation. The latter may both reduce human distinctiveness in relation to animals and mute the concern about human mortality.

Although interpersonal pollution (and, we presume, disgust) is highly developed in Hindu India, the focus of interpersonal disgust in India is foods. In this sense Hindu disgust does rest on core disgust after all. Rules about acceptable and unacceptable foods, formulated in terms of who previously contacted, prepared, or partly consumed a food, are of central importance, and form the principal concrete enactments of the caste system (Marriott, 1968; Appadurai, 1981).

Moral Violation as a Disgust Elicitor and Disgust as One of the Three Other-directed Moral Emotions

Many of the examples for disgust (*ken'o*) listed by American and Japanese subjects involve socio-moral violations that have little obvious connection with either core, animal nature, or interpersonal disgust (Imada, Haidt, McCauley & Rozin, n.d.; Imada, Yamada and Haidt, 1993). We feel that these examples of what we shall call moral disgust can be understood best in the context of a formulation of the nature of moral systems.

Richard Shweder (1990) and Shweder, et al. (1997) have explored moral systems cross-culturally, and suggested that moral ideas and moral arguments around the world tend to fall into three clusters or codes. The first he calls the 'ethics of autonomy', because it takes the autonomy of the individual to be of paramount importance. In this moral code, individuals must always be given the freedom to act on their preferences, and moral dilemmas consist of balancing the rights and welfare of competing autonomous individuals. The second code is called the 'ethics of community', because it takes the community to be of paramount importance, with all of its rules, roles, and traditions. Moral dilemmas in this code typically consist of conflicts between duties or role-based obligations within a hierarchical social structure.

The third code is called the 'ethics of divinity', because it takes spiritual advancement to be of paramount importance. Conflicts within this code focus on the human obligation to strive for closeness to God, physical purity, and the realisation of God within each person, while struggling against the downward forces of material attachment, physical pollution, and animal-like behaviour. Thus Hindu children think that purity violations, such as eating beef or getting a haircut the day after one's father dies, are far more serious moral violations than rights violations such as tearing up the work of another child (Shweder, Mahapatra and Miller, 1987).

We have proposed (Rozin, Haidt and McCauley, 1993; Rozin, Lowery, Imada and Haidt, n.d.) that Shweder's three moral codes map on to what we shall call the three other-directed moral emotions: anger, contempt and disgust. That is, anger is the emotion linked to rights violations, contempt is linked to hierarchy violations, and disgust is linked to purity violations. This prediction was supported in a study in which Japanese, American and Indian subjects read scenarios embodying violations of each of the three Shweder codes. Subjects were presented with an array of anger, contempt and disgust faces and asked to assign each scenario to an emotional reaction. Assignments of scenarios to faces showed the expected linkage of rights, hierarchy, and purity violations with, respectively, anger, contempt, and disgust faces (Rozin, et al., n.d.).

In a related study, Haidt, Koller and Dias (1993) presented violations of the ethics of divinity to lower and upper-class subjects in the United States and Brazil. Scenarios were designed to involve no harm or violation of autonomy, and yet to elicit a sense of disgust: e.g., a family that eats its dead dog, or a man who has sexual relations with a dead animal. The scenarios were considered equally offensive by all groups, but the critical issue was whether the scenarios were considered to be moral violations. In accordance with the dominance of the autonomy/rights code in Western countries, Americans were less inclined to consider disgust violations as immoral (since no one was harmed). Also, upper-class subjects in all settings were less inclined to link disgust and morality. These results, along with our prior discussion, suggest that cultures differ not only in what elicits disgust but in the extent to which disgust elicitors are seen as moral violations. In the event of a moral involvement, however, disgust serves to reinforce the negative attitude to the act.

Historical Perspectives

Our scenario for the cultural evolution of disgust has ontogenetic and historical implications. The ontogenetic implications are simply that one would see a gradual development of disgust elicitors in accordance with the sequence we have laid out – from distaste, to core disgust, to animal-nature disgust, and finally to interpersonal or moral disgust. There are little relevant data at this time.

The historical implications are similar, given that we propose a sequence in cultural evolution. There is some supporting evidence for our scheme, in relation to the particular category of animal nature disgust. There is probably a long history of offense at contact with death, judging for example by Parker's (1983) analysis of miasma and the pollution of death in ancient Greece. We do not know, of course, whether anything like the emotion of disgust was linked to death-pollution at that time. However, it does seem that many aspects of animal nature disgust were not in place in mediæval times in Europe. Norbert Elias' (1978) analysis of the history of manners suggests that mediæval Europeans engaged in many behaviours that would be considered disgusting in modern Western societies. In public eating situations, for example, they ate food from a common pot and returned bitten food to that pot, ate with their hands, and spat at table. Elias accounts for the development of manners as motivated by a desire not to be animal-like: 'it will be shown how people, in the course of the civilizing process, seek to suppress in themselves every characteristic that they feel to be animal'. If we can assume that these behaviours became disgusting, then, following Elias, we can describe disgust as the emotion of civilisation.

Keith Thomas (1983) offers a related analysis of the relation of man to nature in sixteenth to late eighteenth century England. According to Thomas, during this period the uniqueness of humans and their distance from animals became an important part of English sensibilities. Again, we can only presume that these changes were associated with the emergence or enlargement of animal nature disgust. Darwin's major reorientation of views about the relations of animals and humans comes after the period analysed by Thomas. It would be of great interest to analyse the influence of Darwin's ideas about the continuity of humans and animals upon the expression of animal nature disgust. In addition, the decline of organised religion in the last hundred years may have led many people to think about death in a different way, which may in turn have had an effect on the nature or expression of animal nature disgust.

Preadaptation and the Trajectory of Disgust

Our general thesis is that the distaste response, which includes much of the 'programme' (Ekman, 1992) for the emotion of disgust, forms the prototype and basis for disgust. We hold that through a process like evolutionary preadaptation, this programme – an expressive, physiological (nausea), and behavioural rejection system – is attached successively to a variety of things that are offensive within any particular culture. Some of these things, like human faeces, and perhaps contact with death, are likely to be universal, but most are not. Disgust, in this view, becomes the means by which culture can internalise rejection of an offensive object, behaviour, or thought. The phenomenon of contagion, probably originally linked to core disgust, becomes an important component of reactions to the wider range of disgust elicitors, again by a process such as preadaptation.

The process of socialisation in any culture involves acquisition of many values. It is more efficient to have these values internalised than to have to ensure compliance by policing compliance with a rule or law. Disgust accomplishes much of this internalisation of negative values. A good way to prevent traffic with something is to make it an elicitor of disgust.

There are two recent examples of this process in American society. Smoking has, over the last decade, entered into the domain of the immoral, from its prior status as just an undesirable habit (or maybe a desirable one). As this has happened, the manifestations of smoking (e.g., visible cigarette smoke, cigarette stubs or ashes, tobacco stains on teeth) have become disgust elicitors (Rozin and Singh, n.d.).

The process of becoming a vegetarian in modern American culture also illustrates the recruitment of disgust. Some vegetarians adopt their diet almost exclusively for health reasons, others for almost exclusively moral reasons (e.g., animal rights, saving the environment), and many, of course, invoke both types of justification for their vegetarian diet. Comparison of relatively pure 'health' and 'moral' vegetarians indicates that moral vegetarians are much more likely to be disgusted by the prospect of eating meat (Rozin, Markwith and Stoess, 1997). Here we see an example of the 'invocation' of disgust in the service of a moral issue. The vegetarian who is disgusted by meat can be said to have meat avoidance more internalised, and hence to be less tempted to consume meat.

The process of preadaption is central to our analysis. Preadaptation was originally invoked by Ernst Mayr (1960; see also Bock, 1959) as an account of how novel systems could evolve. It seemed unlikely that every small approximation to a novel system would itself be adaptive, and hence subject to selection. Mayr suggested that major evolutionary changes could occur rather rapidly if a system evolved for one purpose was 'borrowed' for another. (Gould and Vrba, 1982, point out that the borrowed structure need not have evolved under natural selection, but could be a neutral trait, and suggest the more general term, exaptation.) A classic example is the evolution of the mammalian middle ear bones (ossicles) from bones in the gill arch. A more familiar example is the human mouth, which clearly evolved as an aperture for processing and handling food (with appropriate adaptations such as tongue and teeth) but which is now shared by the speech output system. The tongue and teeth are essential parts of the articulation of speech sounds, although they did not originally evolve for this purpose.

In order for biological evolutionary preadaptation to occur, the 'pirating system' must have some 'contact' with the original system (Bock, 1959). In the absence of some link, natural selection cannot operate to increase the link. Bock (1959) illustrates the necessity for contact as a prerequisite for preadaptation with the example of a lower jaw bone spur that served as a muscle insertion, which increases in size, makes contact with the upper jaw, and becomes a new jaw artic-ulation. It has been suggested that something like preadaptation (called accessibility) also occurs in individual development, where brain systems involved for one specific purpose become applied in new contexts or domains (Rozin, 1976). For example, it is argued that the auditory speech system linkage in the brain, critically important in spoken language comprehension and production, is partly shared by visual inputs in the process of acquisition of alphabetic writing systems. The phonological segmentation machinery critical for speech perception and production is 'accessed' in the process of learning to read; that is 'how' we come to appreciate that 'bat' has three sounds.

In biological evolution, preadaptation is like mutational variation in that both must wait upon a fortunate set of circumstances. In cul-tural evolution, however, variation can be intentionally produced and so can preadaptation. An individual, group or culture can put ideas in contact in ways that will serve as a preadaptation for cultural selection. We can recognise, for example, that the calculator and typewriter, if combined, could make a computer, or that the same principle used in a motorcycle, if enlarged and modified, could transport large loads in things as do trucks and cars. The history of technology (Girifalco, 1991) is, in substantial part, a history of pre-adaptations. Similarly, it is our claim that the sequence of evolution via preadaptation that we have presented for disgust represents a common sequence in cultural evolution.

Our analysis suggests that the major event in the cultural evolution of disgust is the expansion or replacement of meanings and elicitors, with the output side of the emotion programme largely intact. This is not to say that there have been no changes on the output side. Recent studies of the facial expressions related to recognition of disgust suggest that there is a difference in prototypical expressions associated with different types of disgust (Rozin, Lowery and Ebert, 1994; critical studies on the production of disgust faces to different elicitors have yet to be done). Thus, distaste associated with bitter or sour tastes seems to be primarily related to lip pressing and purses, neither hallmarks of disgust. The gaping response, characteristic (along with the lip press and purse; Rosenstein and Oster, 1988) of infant responses to bad tastes seems primarily associated with two types of elicitors: oral irritation from high temperature or irritants like chilli peppers, and core disgust food entities such as rotten foods. On the other hand, animal nature, interpersonal and moral disgust are most associated with a raising of the upper lip. It is perhaps not accidental that this dominant expression of elaborated disgust has no obvious function in expelling foods or odours, but is rather linked to the mammalian upper lip raise associated with baring of the teeth. Disgust shares, in this respect, a facial expression also commonly seen in the anger face. As disgust approaches the moral domain, it seems to become more involved with an expression associated with another moral emotion.

Our conception of disgust is incomplete and undeveloped. We feel it is appropriate to at least call attention to a different, but somewhat related idea. It comes from Mary Douglas' (1966) analysis of the concept of pollution. Douglas sees pollution as an expression of 'matter out of place', that is anomalousness or uncanniness. She holds that the human psyche is offended by things that do not fit into accepted schemes, and such entities are polluting (and perhaps, disgusting). It is clear that anomaly, often manifested as deformity (such as amputated limb stumps, absence or unusual conformation of facial features) is a substantial elicitor of disgust. This falls roughly under our more limited category of body envelope violations. However, it is also clear that anomaly is neither a necessary nor a sufficient condition for the elicitation of disgust.

We are just at the beginning of understanding the cultural differentiation of disgust. We have suggested that important cultural values will correspond to notable variations in what is found offensive, immoral and disgusting in particular cultures. Thus, we have proposed that issues of social management may enter the disgust domain in Japan, and issues of interpersonal contact and morality may become primary in the expression of disgust in Hindu India. Whatever the validity of these particular suggestions, we are confident that the study of disgust will be useful in understanding cultural development and cultural variation. Disgust is culture's most effective means to enforce a prohibition.

Acknowledgement

We thank the Whitehall Foundation for supporting some of the research reported in this paper and the preparation of this chapter.

References

Angyal, A. (1941) Disgust and related aversions, *Journal of Abnormal and Social Psychology*, 36: 393-412

Appadurai, A. (1981) Gastro-politics in Hindu South Asia, *American Ethnologist*, 8: 494-511

Becker, E. (1973) *The Denial of Death*, Free Press, New York

Bock, W.J. (1959) Preadaptation and multiple evolutionary pathways, *Evolution*, 13: 194-211

Chiva, M. (1985) *Le Doux et l'Amer*, Presses Universitaires de France, Paris

Darwin, C. R. (1872) *The Expression of Emotions in Man and Animals*, John Murray, London (Reprinted by University Of Chicago Press, 1965)

DesPres, T. (1976) *The Survivor*, Oxford University Press

Douglas, M. (1966) *Purity and Danger*, Routledge & Kegan Paul, London

Ekman, P. (1992) An argument for basic emotions, *Cognition and Emotion*, 6: 169-200

Elias, N. (1939/1978) *The History of Manners: the Civilizing Process* Vol. I (E. Jephcott, Trans.), Pantheon Books, New York (Original work published 1939)

Fallon, A.E., and Rozin, P. (1983) The psychological bases of food rejections by humans, *Ecology of Food and Nutrition*, 13: 15-26

Frazer, J.G. (1890/1959) *The Golden Bough: A Study in Magic and Religion*, Macmillan, New York (reprint of 1922 abridged edition, T.H.Gaster (ed.), original work published, 1890).

Girifalco, L.A. (1991) *The Dynamics of Technological Change*, Van Nostrand Reinhold, New York

Gould, S.J. and Vrba, E.S. (1982) Exaptation: a missing term in the science of form, *Paleobiology*, 8: 4-15

Grill, H.J., and Norgren, R. (1977) The taste reactivity test, I: oro-facial responses to gustatory stimuli in neurologically normal rats, *Brain Research*, 143: 263-79

Haidt, J., Koller, S.H., and Dias, M.G. (1993) Disgust, disrespect and moral judgment in the U.S. and Brazil, *Journal of Personality and Social Psychology*, 65: 613-28

Haidt, J., McCauley, C.R., and Rozin, P. (in press) A scale to measure disgust sensitivity, *Personality and Individual Difference*, 16: 701-713

Haidt, J., Rozin, P., McCauley, C.R., and Imada, S. (in press) Body, psyche and culture: The relationship between disgust and morality, in G. Misra (ed.), *The Cultural Construction of Social Cognition*

Imada, S., Haidt, J., McCauley, C., & Rozin, P. (n.d.) *A Scale for the Measurement of Disgust in Japan* (unpublished m.s.)

Imada, S., Yamada, Y., & Haidt, J. (1993) The differences of Ken'o (disgust) experiences for Japanese and American students, *Studies in the Humanities and Sciences*, 34, Hiroshima Shudo University

Lakoff, G. and Johnson, M. (1980) *Metaphors We Live By*, Chicago University Press

Leach, E. (1964) Anthropological aspects of language: Animal categories and verbal abuse, in E. Lenneberg (ed.), *New Directions in the Study of Language*, Cambridge, Massachusetts M.I.T. Press, 23-64

Markus, H.R. and Kitayama, S. (1991) Culture and self: implications for cognition, emotion and motivation, *Psychological Review*, 98: 224-53

Marriott, M. (1968) Caste ranking and food transactions: A matrix analysis, in M. Singer and B.S. Cohn (eds.), *Structure and Change in Indian society*, Aldine, Chicago, 133-71

Mauss, M. (1902/1972) *A General Theory of Magic* (R. Brain, Trans.), W.W. Norton, New York (original work published 1902, Esquisse d'une theorie generale de la magie, *L'Annee Sociologique*, 1902-1903)

Mayr, E. (1960) The emergence of evolutionary novelties, in S. Tax (eds.), *Evolution after Darwin: the Evolution of Life*, Vol. 1, University of Chicago Press

McCauley, C.R., Rozin, P., and Markwith, M. (n.d.) *Aversion to Interpersonal Contact with Strangers: a Two Component Analysis* (unpublished m.s.)

Meigs, A.S. (1984) *Food, Sex, and Pollution: A New Guinea Religion*, Rutgers University Press, New Brunswick, New Jersey

Nemeroff, C., and Rozin, P. (1989) 'You are what you eat': Applying the demand-free 'impressions' technique to an unacknowledged belief, *Ethos: Journal of Psychological Anthropology,* 17: 50-69

Nemeroff, C., and Rozin, P. (1994) The contagion concept in adult thinking in the United States: Transmission of germs and interpersonal influence, *Ethos: Journal of Psychological Anthropology,* 22: 158-86

Parker, R. (1983) *Miasma: Pollution and Purification in Early Greek Religion*, Oxford University Press

Petó, E. (1936) Contribution to the development of smell feeling, *British Journal of Medical Psychology*, 15: 314-320

Rosenstein, D. and Oster, H. (1988) Differential facial responses to four basic tastes in newborns, *Child Development*, 59: 1,555-68

Rozin, P. (1976) The evolution of intelligence and access to the cognitive unconscious, in J.A. Sprague and A.N. Epstein (eds.), *Progress in Psychobiology and Physiological Psychology*, Academic Press, New York, 6: 245-80

Rozin, P., Fallon, A.E. and Augustoni-Ziskind, M. (1986) The child's conception of food: development of categories of accepted and rejected substances, *Journal of Nutrition Education* 18: 75-81

Rozin, P., Haidt, J. and McCauley, C.R. (1993) Disgust, in M. Lewis and J. Haviland (eds.), *Handbook of Emotions*, Guilford, New York, 575-94

Rozin, P., Hammer, L., Oster, H., Horowitz, T. and Marmara, V. (1986) The child's conception of food: differentiation of categories of rejected substances in the 1.4 to 5 year age range, *Appetite*, 7: 141-51

Rozin, P., Lowery, L., & Ebert, R. (1994) Varieties of disgust faces and the structure of disgust, *Journal of Personality and Social Psychology*, 66: 870-81

Rozin, P., Lowery, L., Imada, S. and Haidt, J. (n.d.) *The Moral/Emotion (CAD) Hypothesis: a Mapping Between the Other-Directed Moral Emotions: Disgust, Contempt, and Anger; and Shweder's Three Universal Moral Codes* (unpublished m.s.)

Rozin, P., Markwith, M. and McCauley, C.R. (1994) The nature of aversion to indirect contact with other persons: AIDS aversion as a composite of aversion to strangers, infection, moral taint and misfortune, *Journal of Abnormal Psychology*, 103: 495-504

Rozin, P., Markwith, M., and Stoess, C. (1977) Moralization: Becoming a vegetarian, the conversion of preferences into values and the recruitment of disgust. *Psychological Science*, 8: 67-73

Rozin, P., Millman, L. and Nemeroff, C. (1986) Operation of the laws of sympathetic magic in disgust and other domains, *Journal of Personality and Social Psychology*, 50: 703-712

Rozin, P., and Nemeroff, C.J. (1990) The laws of sympathetic magic: A psychological analysis of similarity and contagion, in J. Stigler, G. Herdt and R.A. Shweder (eds.) *Cultural Psychology: Essays on Comparative Human Development*, Cambridge University Press, 205-32

Rozin, P. and Singh, L. (n.d.) *The Moralization of Cigarette Smoking in America* (submitted ms.)

Shweder, R.A. (1990) In defense of moral realism: reply to Gabennesch, *Child Development*, 61: 2,060-7

Shweder, R.A., Mahapatra, M. and Miller, J.G. (1987) Culture and moral development, in J. Kagan & S. Lamb (eds.), *The Emergence of Moral Concepts in Young Children*, University of Chicago Press, 1-82

Shweder, R.A., Much, N.C., Mahapatra, M. and Park, L. (1997) The 'big three' of morality (autonomy, community, divinity), and the 'big three' explanations of suffering, in A. Brandt and P. Rozin (eds.), *Morality and Health*, Routledge, New York, 119-69

Steiner, J.E. (1979) Human facial expressions in response to taste and smell stimulation, in H.W. Reese and L.P. Lipsitt (eds.), *Advances in Child Development and Behaviour*, Academic Press, New York, 13: 257-95

Tambiah, S.J. (1969) Animals are good to think and good to prohibit, *Ethnology*, 8: 423-59

Thomas, K. (1983) *Man and the Natural World*, Pantheon Books, New York

Tylor, E.B. (1871/1974) *Primitive Culture: Researches into the Development of Mythology, Philosophy, Religion, Art and Custom*, Gordon Press, New York (Original work published 1871)

Wronska, J. (1990) Disgust in relation to emotionality, extraversion, psychoticism and imagery abilities, in P. Drenth, J. Sergeant, and R. Taken (eds.), *European Perspectives in Psychology*, Vol. 1, John Wiley & Sons, Chichester, U.K.

7. WILD PLANTS AS FAMINE FOODS
FOOD CHOICE UNDER CONDITIONS OF SCARCITY

Rebecca Huss-Ashmore and *Susan L. Johnston*

Throughout history, famine and food shortage have been salient features of subsistence and peasant societies. Types of food shortage reported for pre-industrial groups vary from mild seasonal shortfalls in staple foods to occasional widespread and severe hunger. While in recent decades we have seen famines restricted to Africa and parts of Asia, there is probably no geographic region that has not experienced severe food shortage at some time in the past (Robson, 1981). As food shortage is so widespread in subsistence-oriented societies, such groups have developed strategies for coping with scarcity. These strategies can be seen as part of the overall adaptive repertoire of pre-industrial populations, and range from food sharing and reliance on less preferred foods to permanent migration and the sale of land and livestock.

One of the most frequently reported strategies for dealing with scarcity, whether short or long term, is the collecting and consumption of wild plants. Even for societies such as those of foragers, where wild plants are part of the normal diet, there is an increase in the range of plants exploited when staple foods are scarce. For many cultivators, wild plants that are condiments and medicines in normal times make increasing nutritional contributions when food supplies fail.

Despite the importance of wild foods as famine strategies, there has been little systematic research on the topic, and little is known about the psychological, cultural, or biological factors that govern their choice and use. Etkin (1986; 1993) and others (e.g., Iwu, 1986; Keith and Armelagos, 1983) have explored the medicinal role of wild plant foods, including cognitive features involved in medicinal plant choice. Further, Johns (1986; Johns and Keen, 1986) has outlined chemical factors that influence the use of wild plants as potential cultigens. While plant knowledge and selection criteria are part of a group's adaptive pattern, the calculus of choice involved in famine foods has not been systematically investigated. This paper sets out models that have been used to explain food choice and wild plant use and evaluates their relevance for choice of famine foods. It first examines models of choice based on taste and other hedonic factors, and then presents alternative models that incorporate social and ecological factors in plant food selection. Ethnographic examples of famine food use from Africa and aboriginal North America are used to illustrate the costs and benefits of wild plant use under conditions of food scarcity.

Famine Foods as Coping Strategy

There is a growing literature on the coping strategies employed by different populations faced with regular or occasional deficits in food supply. Most of these studies are concerned either with seasonal hunger or with famine, and with the hierarchy of responses to these different types of shortage. Recent food crises in Africa have made it the focus for much of the discussion on hunger (Glantz, 1986; Hansen and McMillan, 1986; Huss-Ashmore and Katz, 1989), but food stress has also been reported for many areas of south and southeast Asia, as well as for historical Europe, east Asia, the Pacific, and aboriginal North America. In general, short-term and predictable food shortage is dealt with by types of self insurance, such as storage, seasonal labour migration, exchange between households, food rationing, and increased collecting of wild foods. If shortage persists or becomes severe, these precautions may be insufficient, and more extreme measures may be required. Watts (1983) and Corbett (1988) note that low cost, reversible responses give way to high cost, irreversible measures with prolonged or more severe food deficit, as productive assets are increasingly pledged, eaten, or sold. Changes in diet, including lowered consumption levels and reliance on foraged foods, are preventive strategies that preserve household assets, increasing the probability of economic recovery once the crisis is past (Corbett, 1988).

The reliance on wild foods to supplement and extend household food supplies is one of the most widely reported hunger strategies, and emergency plant foods have been identified for every continent. Although wild foods include foods of animal origin, including mammals, fish, reptiles, birds, and insects (Cowen, 1992; Dufour, 1987; 1992), wild plants have the greatest dietary importance. Plant organs and products commonly consumed as emergency foods include:

1. rhizomes, roots, and tubers,
2. leaves of perennial plants,
3. pulp of fruits of woody perennials, and
4. seeds of certain wild grasses (Irvine, 1952).

In addition, buds, stems, bark, gums, saps, and flowers may be eaten, although less widely or in smaller amounts.

The nutritional importance of these different plant products varies by ecological zone and with the usual subsistence orientation of the consumers (Huss-Ashmore and Johnston, 1994). Roots and seeds appear to be especially important in arid areas such as the Kalahari and the American Southwest, especially for foragers, while barks and lichens have been more widely used in temperate areas. Potatoes and other tubers, freeze-dried to remove the bitter alkaloids, are a traditional famine food strategy in the South American highlands (NRC, 1989), while tree gums and saps are reported as famine foods in arid regions of aboriginal Australia (Levitt, 1981) and southern Africa (Hitchcock, 1989). Edible leaves and stems of both annual and perennial plants appear to be important famine foods across a variety of societies in different ecological zones. Their use is widely reported for agricultural societies in all regions of Africa, as condiments in normal times, as relishes or side dishes during the growing season, and as staple foods during times of crop failure (Grivetti et al., 1987; Huss-Ashmore and Johnston, 1994). In addition, they are reported as emergency foods from Nepal (Regmi, 1982; Malla et al., 1982), India (Singh and Arora, 1978), China (Read, 1977), and aboriginal North America (Kindscher, 1987; Kuhnlein and Turner, 1991).

The biological importance of famine foods should be a function of both their nutritional properties and the non-nutritional results of their ingestion. The ability of wild plants to provide sufficient energy and other nutrients is obviously critical for survival during periods of food shortage, but other aspects of plant biochemistry are also potentially important for human adaptation. Johns (1986; 1990), Jackson (1991), and Stahl (1984) have all argued that wild plants have had a significant impact on human evolution through the ingestion of secondary plant compounds (allelochemicals). These compounds include alkaloids, glycosides, phenolics, and non-protein amino acids, among others. As part of the plants' own defences against predators, many of these compounds are both bitter and toxic. Successful adaptation by human populations would require either recognition and avoidance of toxic plants, or biological and cultural methods of detoxification. During famine, when choice of foodstuffs is constrained, effective detoxification should become especially important. Thus both selection and processing strategies contribute to the effectiveness of a population's response to food shortage.

Food Choice During Scarcity

While there is an extensive literature on food choice and preference, there is little data on the ways in which humans make choices during scarcity. Even during periods of shortage, it is clear that not everything edible is eaten, and it is only with the threat of true starvation that productive resources (horses, dogs), culturally proscribed food sources (carrion, other humans) and non-nutritive items (wood, leather) will be used (Hitchcock, 1989; Steegman, 1983). As in other situations, hedonic factors may be involved in choice of famine foods, but as famine progresses, taste preferences are likely to be modified by notions of nutritive value. In extreme situations, perceived nutritional value of a food, or even the feeling of fullness it provides, may override bad taste, known toxicity, cultural proscription, and even personal feelings of disgust. Thus models explaining food choice under scarcity need to include cultural and biological factors not usually considered for situations of food abundance. We examine here a series of frameworks that have been used to explain food choice, in the light of their usefulness for the study of famine foods, especially wild plant foods.

Psychobiological models

Much of the work on the psychobiology of food choice is concerned with the role of taste and other senses in determining food preference. The question addressed in much of this research is the degree to which food choice is based on innate or genetic factors, and the nutritional wisdom that food choice reflects. Thus research in this area has addressed the taste sensitivity of newborns, the neurological basis of feeding and satiety, and the ability of omnivores to choose nutritionally balanced diets from an array of available foods (Booth, 1982). In general, few innate taste preferences have been demonstrated for omnivores, and most of the variability seen in stable food preferences is attributed to learning. Both rats and humans show an innate preference for sweetness and an innate distaste for bitterness (Beauchamp, 1981; Rozin, 1990), but can be conditioned to like or dislike a broad range of flavours. Among the specific hungers studied, only the preference for salt has been unequivocally linked to the innate recognition of a state of nutrient deficiency (Rozin and Schulkin, 1990). Other long-term food preferences are presumed to reflect the animal's post-ingestive experience, that is, whether eating a particular food in the past has made it feel good or bad. Such learning appears possible even with long lag times between ingestion and consequences (Barker, 1982). The preference for energy-dense foods such as fats and complex carbohydrates (starch) is probably learned in relation to the feelings of satiety that they invoke (Booth, 1982; Drewnowski and Greenwood, 1983).

Social factors, i.e., what conspecifics eat, also influence learned food preferences. Both rats and primates eat new foods more readily if these are eaten by others of their species (Galef, 1988), and this learning seems to be mediated largely by smell. For humans, social and cultural factors influence which foods children are exposed to and therefore learn to prefer (P. Rozin, 1982). Social factors also influence preference directly, in that children like foods more if they perceive that they are enjoyed by their peers (Birch, 1986).

Both innate taste preference and learned food preference or avoidance should be relevant to the selection of wild plant foods. Innate taste sensitivities are presumably adaptive, in that sweet substances are usually nutritive, and bitter ones often toxic. Previous experiences with wild plant products, used in normal times as food or as medicine, would also provide information on the expected consequences of ingestion. Many of the wild plants used during hunger periods have parts with medicinal or culinary uses (flavourings, thickening agents). Others are normally eaten by children as snacks (Fleuret, 1979; 1986), and such childhood dietary exploration may provide background knowledge for selection of emergency foods. Flavour memories and taste aversions learned between the ages of six and twelve seem especially tenacious (Barker, 1982), so that childhood foraging would be an important means of gaining knowledge about the potentially edible resources in the environment. Familiarity with a range of wild foods should further increase their acceptability by lessening the neophobia, or distrust of novel foods, reported for omnivores (Rozin, 1990). On the other hand, knowledge of plant toxicity and foods to be avoided could also be reinforced by this process.

Cultural models

While trial and error learning during childhood is likely to be important in wild plant knowledge and use, most of an individual's store of environmental knowledge is likely to come from other people. Social factors are important in dietary selection even in rats, and are probably paramount for humans. Etkin (1986) has emphasised the importance of cultural encoding of wild plant knowledge for the operation of ethnomedical systems. She points out that the cultural meanings and values ascribed to food plants by any given population will affect their patterns of use or avoidance. These meanings include ideas about the intrinsic qualities of the plant, its relationship to the cosmological order of the society, and its effect, through magical or material means, on human health and functioning (Etkin 1986). Thus societies with humoural systems of medicine may select plants as either food or medicine based on their ability to maintain or restore humoural balance. Similarly, plant choice may be based on the belief that material and visible qualities of the plant signify its appropriate use. The use of plants with milky sap or latex as galactagogues and the use of phallomorphic roots as aphrodisiacs exemplify this principle (Ferro-Luzzi, 1980; Jerome et al., 1980).

There is limited systematic information on the application of such ethnobiological principles to plants used as food. Humoural principles in diet have received the most attention, with hot-cold and yin-yang dichotomies widely reported to affect food choice. Principles of traditional Chinese medicine are certainly reflected in diet (Helman, 1990), and hot-cold beliefs are thought to affect the intake of protein, vitamins, and minerals in populations from Latin America to South Asia and Malaysia (Ferro-Luzzi, 1980; Logan, 1972; McKay, 1980; Wilson, 1980). Katz (1987) and E. Rozin (1982) have suggested that cuisine, or the cultural rules for food preparation and consumption, may play an adaptive role by encoding information on the most nutritious or medically efficacious use of foodstuffs. Both food processing (cooking, fermenting, leaching, etc.) and the ways in which foods are combined in dishes and meals can affect nutritional and pharmacological qualities of the diet (Johns and Kubo, 1988; Etkin, 1993). Timing of plant use may be biologically important and may also be encoded through cuisine. Etkin and Ross (1991) have argued that the seasonal use of anti-malarial plants in the diet of the Hausa may have an important role in mitigating malarial outbreaks.

Culture provides rules not only for what is to be eaten, but who is to eat it. Within any culture, certain foods are deemed appropriate for some categories of people and not for others. The most extreme examples of this are seen in food proscriptions or 'taboos' that limit the intake of specific foods for groups of people based on their age, sex, or social, reproductive, or ritual status (de Garine and Hladik, 1990; Ferro-Luzzi, 1980). Alternatively, such rules may operate to provide extra food or foraging opportunities for nutritionally vulnerable individuals, such as new mothers, children, and the elderly (Huss-Ashmore and Glantz, 1993). For example, primiparous mothers among the Ntomba of Zaire receive extra food during the period of postpartum seclusion (Pagezy, 1990), and variants of this practice can be found among southern Bantu groups as well (Miller and Huss-Ashmore, 1989).

The degree to which these principles apply to choice of emergency foods is not clear. Cuisine is likely to be important, at least in the early stages of food scarcity, in that the cultural rules for preparation and serving of staple foods can be applied to novel foods used during emergencies. For example, methods for preparing cassava and cultivated yams can be used to detoxify wild yams and other tubers eaten during food shortage (Irvine, 1952). Johns (1986; 1990) further suggests that the widespread practice of geophagy during famine may be designed to produce a feeling of fullness when food is unavailable, but is also an efficient way of detoxifying wild plants used during food crises. The use of clays as condiments with certain highly toxic foods (e.g., solanine – and tomatine-rich potatoes in the Andes) is thus a culinary practice that should enhance survival for populations that practise it.

The cultural rules governing access to food may operate either to protect vulnerable groups from hunger or to exclude them from emergency food sources. The poor have little resilience, either economically or nutritionally, and are often the first to migrate during famine (Corbett, 1988). Similarly, children and the elderly show higher mortality when shortage is severe. De Garine (1993; de Garine and Koppert, 1988) shows the ambiguous position of the elderly among the Massa and Mussey of Cameroon. No longer economically active, they may have little support within the community, and may even be used as tasters for potentially toxic famine foods. On the other hand, as marginal persons, they are allowed to eat foods thought inappropriate or disgusting by other groups of people. De Garine (1993) attributes the vulnerable position of the elderly in these societies to the breakdown of traditional reciprocity. Where the elderly still act as repositories of valuable wild food knowledge, their opportunities for survival during famine should be enhanced.

Ecological and evolutionary models

The ecological tradition within anthropology has emphasised the interaction between human populations and their environments.

While a number of authors have proposed ecological models to explain diet or nutritional status, few of these have addressed food choice. For example, May (1961; May and McLellan, 1970) has written extensively on the ecology of malnutrition in different geographical regions, and Jerome et al. (1980) and Brown (1986) have proposed ecological models for the study of food and nutrition. In all of these, diet is influenced not only by the physical environment, but also by food production technology, social organisation, and cultural systems. Food choice is not considered explicitly in any of these models, but is assumed to be a product of food availability and cultural definitions of what is appropriate for different groups.

In one of the few models to address choice directly, Krondl and Lau (1982) envisage food choice as the interface between food availability and the decision to choose among foods. Food use is determined by factors intrinsic to the individual (age, sex, genetic heritage), exogenous factors (culture, society, economy), and perception (beliefs, prestige, convenience, taste, familiarity, etc.) This framework emphasises the operation of psychological factors within a social environment; physical and biotic environments are not considered, except as they might operate through economic factors. In contrast, Johns (1990) emphasises the interaction between humans and their biotic and chemical environments, stressing the potential evolutionary consequences of plant food choice. His model of chemical ecology posits that humans seek to maximise the beneficial effects of foods selected and minimise potential toxic effects. Natural selection is assumed to have produced physiological and behavioural mechanisms, especially language and technology, that allow humans to deal successfully with environmental chemicals.

The idea of maximising benefit and minimising costs of food choice is elaborated further in models from behavioural ecology. Optimal foraging models are especially important for considering the selection and use of wild plants. These models share the underlying assumption that organisms will behave as if they are optimising some fitness related currency, such as energy or nutrient capture (Kaplan and Hill, 1992). Foods sought should therefore be ranked by their profitability (net nutrient gains divided by handling time) and not by their food value alone. As the abundance of highly profitable resources decreases, both the time spent searching for foods and the number of different types used are expected to increase (Pyke, 1984).

Food availability and the costs and benefits of foraging are concepts especially important to the understanding of famine food choice. By definition, scarcity reduces the availability of food resources. While extreme food shortage may reduce the availability of everything edible, in most cases, shortage is perceived as a lack of preferred foods (Ogbu, 1973), i.e., those that are not only familiar but that are palatable and dense in preferred nutrients such as fat or protein. Up to a point, greater effort should be made to procure preferred foods, but when the opportunity cost of that strategy becomes too high, a shift should be made to less palatable or less 'profitable' resources.

We have proposed a framework for studying famine foods that takes into account the adaptive strategies of the plants used, as well as the costs and benefits of their use (Huss-Ashmore and Johnston, 1994). The availability of plant resources during periods of shortage is partly a function of how well those resources are adapted to environmental conditions. Relevant plant adaptations include their ability to withstand heat, cold, drought, flooding, wind, and a variety of pests and predators. In general, indigenous wild plants are better adapted to local environmental conditions than are introduced cultigens. Human populations that rely on wild plants during periods of environmental stress are merely taking advantage of the superior adaptation of indigenous species.

Plant strategies for dealing with environmental hazards include storage structures, climate resistant architecture, biochemical defence against predators, and changes in life history tactics. Thus plants subjected to regular drought or cold may show seasonal dormancy, rapid energy cycling, extensive root networks, woody and waxy surfaces, subterranean stems and roots, and a variety of other organs for storage of water and nutrients (Nabhan, 1989; Solbrig and Orians, 1977). In addition, they frequently exhibit tough, fibrous textures and bitter tastes or toxins that discourage predators. Emergency plant foods are therefore likely to be the products of well defended plants and those whose storage strategies allow them to survive where more fragile plants could not. However, the costs associated with using these plants may be high; they are often sparsely distributed and low in nutrient density. Furthermore, cellulose and toxins may require extensive processing to make them edible or even minimally palatable.

We suggest, therefore, that emergency plant foods may be chosen according to a calculus that weighs potential benefits (perceived nutritional value, satiety, taste) against perceived costs (time and energy to collect and process, probable toxicity). If food shortage persists, less palatable foods and those with higher time costs and greater health risk should be increasingly used. Under these conditions, an increase in diet breadth, i.e., the variety of resources used, should be seen. While this model has not been empirically tested, ethnographic data from Africa and from aboriginal North America suggest that progressively costly food choice strategies may be employed as scarcity increases.

Ethnographic Examples

Accounts of wild plant use are available from all regions of Africa, but their use as emergency foods is documented primarily for the arid and semi-arid savannas and savanna woodlands of West Africa, Southern Africa, and East Africa including Ethiopia and the Sudan. All these areas are characterised by sparse and unpredictable rainfall and by marked wet/dry seasonality. While the number of wild plant foods used is large, roots, leaves, and fruits are the most commonly used products (Irvine, 1952). Roots and other starchy underground organs are sought for their carbohydrate content and satiety value, while leaves provide considerable protein and calcium and some fat. Fruits provide sugars and some vitamins, but are often sour, small, and widely dispersed.

Irvine (1952) notes the costs involved in famine foods used in West Africa. He points out that a variety of roots, tubers, and rhizomes are used as emergency foods in this area, and that many of these contain toxins. Cassava is probably the best known of these and is regularly used during lean seasons as a substitute for grain (Watts, 1983). In addition, roots and rhizomes of lilies, legumes, and aroids are collected and eaten after processing to remove bitter or toxic compounds. During severe droughts, wild yams are also used, despite their content of dioscorine, a potent nervous system paralytic. The process of detoxification involves peeling, boiling, slicing, and pounding the tubers, then soaking them in running or salt water for up to three days. Despite this, the wild cluster yam has been blamed for a number of deaths (Corkill, 1948).

Other toxic plants eaten by African populations during severe food shortage include succulents such as *Euphorbia candelabrum*, a relative of the prickly pear (Rahmato, 1991), wild cucumber (Quin, 1959), and the seeds of leguminous trees (*Acacia albida*) and a number of wild grasses (Scudder 1971). Seeds known to be poisonous are usually soaked and boiled, but despite processing, seeds of *Boscia sensgule* have been blamed for a number of child deaths in the Sudan (Sukkary-Stolba, 1989). Thus processing costs and health risks appear high for a number of plants used under famine conditions.

Increased foraging time and decreased nutrient density also appear to characterise foods used as shortage worsens. For example, de Garine and Koppert (1988) note that grass seeds are gathered by the Massa and Mussey only in situations of true hunger, in that gathering and pounding the tiny seeds is a time consuming task. Low nutrient density is especially characteristic of starvation foods. Riley and Brokensha (1988) report the use of acacia and baobab bark by the Mbeere of Kenya during severe famine conditions, while Sukkary-Stolba (1989) lists peanut shells and grain stored by termites as starvation foods in the Sudan. For the Tyua of Botswana, starvation foods include tree gums, leaves, bark, and old animal skins and leather (Hitchcock et al., 1989).

In contrast to Africa, emergency foods for aboriginal North America are known primarily from ethnohistorical accounts. Shortages seem to have been occasioned by severe winters, seasonal or more extended droughts, floods, and more long-term processes such as game depletion and forced resettlement (Steegman, 1983; Steward, 1938). The greater variety of ecological conditions led to a greater variety of plant foods used than is currently the case in Africa: reported categories include algae, lichens, and ferns, as well as flowering plants. Plant parts used most prominently during scarcity included perennial greens, bark and cambium, fruits, roots and seeds (Kuhnlein and Turner, 1991).

As in the African case, North American famine foods contained a number of species that were highly toxic. Lichens were one of the most widespread emergency foods in northern areas, and one of the most likely to cause digestive upsets. They contain complex polysaccharides and are often bitter; many also contain the toxins, vulpinic and usnic acids (Airaksinen et al., 1986). Indigenous strategies to improve taste and digestibility included soaking in water or in an alkaline solution (water and ash) and boiling. Reindeer moss, one of the more toxic lichens used, was sometimes collected from caribou rumens in a partially digested state, which decreased its toxicity (Kuhnlein and Turner, 1991). Acorns were used as a staple on the California coast, but were also used as a famine food in the interior of the continent (Steegman, 1983); even after repeated leaching, the flour of many acorn species remains bitter due to tannic and other acids. Other poisonous plants used during emergencies were algae, used in coastal areas, the root of prairie turnip, eaten on the plains, and skunk cabbage, eaten in the Pacific north-west (Kuhnlein and Turner, 1991). Toxicity has also been suggested for the cambium of the bittersweet vine used throughout the Great Lakes region (Jones, 1965).

While there is little reliable information on starvation conditions in aboriginal North America, several accounts indicate the use of foods with decreasing nutritional value or density as shortage became severe. Lichens and barks, some of the most common famine foods, are relatively low in energy, although they contain some carbohydrate and minerals. In addition, among the forest Algonkian peoples, last resort foods included hide (clothing, skins, snowshoe webbing), tree bark, entrails and carrion, and dogs (Steegman, 1983). One report from the upper Missouri River during the early eighteenth century lists a sequence of resort for the Assiniboin when no meat was available: dried berries and roots, rawhide scrapings boiled with rose hips, grease extracted from pounded bones, and finally, dogs and horses (Kindscher, 1987). In these cases, the cost of famine foods clearly included the cost of eating productive resources, as horses and dogs were necessary for hunting.

In a recent study of drought response among the Mountain Pima, Laferriere (1992) showed that diet breadth increased as cultivated crops failed. The most important wild plants used were the pads and fruits of the prickly pear (*Opuntia spp.*) and a variety of wild greens (mostly *Amaranthus,' Portulaca* and *Chenopodium*). Less preferred species used included agave stalks and manzanilla berries; the more toxic local acorns and cebollin bulbs were reported as used in past famines, but both require extensive processing and are not currently used. Wage labour and livestock sales provided cash for the purchase of emergency foods, which served as a substitute for the less palatable wild resources.

Conclusion

Anthropologists interested in human adaptability have generally agreed that the basic adaptive tasks of any population include the avoidance of stressors and the procurement of critical resources. While there is ample research on environmental stressors and responses to these (Frisancho, 1979; Little and Haas, 1989), work on the adaptive aspects of resource procurement has only begun (Hames, 1992; Kaplan and Hill, 1992; Smith 1983). Strategies for acquiring and using food resources under conditions of scarcity are still poorly understood, although recent studies of seasonal ecology (e.g., Laferriere, 1992; Little et al., 1992; Pyke and Winterbauer, 1993) should improve this situation. The widespread occurrence of food shortage in subsistence societies suggests that such strategies are part of the human evolutionary heritage. Including famine foods within an ecological and evolutionary framework should therefore be a research priority, in that fitness is most likely to be affected when food is scarce. The ability to deal with scarcity successfully should involve biological and behavioural responses, including taste preferences and flavour memories, cultural rules for food choice and preparation, and strategies to weigh the changing costs and benefits of resource procurement. Models incorporating these multiple dimensions will be necessary for understanding the role that wild plants play in human adaptation to recurring food stress.

References

Airaksinen, M.M., Peura P.L., Ala-Possi-Salokangas, L., Antere, S., Lukkarinen, J., Saikkonen, M. and Stenback, F. (1986) Toxicity of plant material used as emergency food during famines in Finland, *Journal of Ethnopharmacology*, 18: 273-96

Barker, L.M. (1982) Building memories for foods, in L.M. Barker (ed.), *The Psychobiology of Human Food Selection*, AVI Publishing Co. Westport, CT, 85-100

Beauchamp, G.K. (1981) Ontogenesis of taste preference, in D. Walcher and N. Kretchmer (eds.), *Food, Nutrition, and Evolution*, Masson, New York, 49-57

Birch, L.L. (1986) Children's food preferences: developmental patterns and environmental influences, in G. Whitehurst and R. Vasta (eds.), *Annals of Child Development*, JAI, Greenwich, CT, 171-208

Booth, D.A. (1982) How nutritional effects of foods can influence people's dietary choices, in L.M. Barker (ed.), *The Psychobiology of Human Food Selection*, AVI Publishing Co. Westpoint, CT, 67-84

Brown, A.B. (1986) Nutritional anthropology: the community focus, in S.A. Quandt and C. Ritenbaugh (eds.), *Training Manual in Nutritional Anthropology*, American Anthropological Association, Washington, DC, 41-59

Corbett, J. (1988) Famine and household coping strategies, *World Development* 16(9): 1,099-112

Corkill, N.L. (1948) The poisonous wild cluster yam, *Dioscorea dumetorum Pax*, as a famine food in the Anglo-Egyptian Sudan, *Annals of Tropical Medicine and Parasitology*, 42: 278-87

Cowen, R. (1992) Butterflies in their stomachs, *Science News*, 141(15): 236

De Garine, I. (1993) Coping strategies in case of hunger of the most vulnerable groups among the Massa and Mussey of Northern Cameroon, *GeoJournal*, 30: 159-66

De Garine, I. and C.M. Hladik (1990) Nutritional concepts: perception, food prohibitions and prescriptions, in C.M. Hladik, S. Bahuchet, and

I. de Garine, (eds.), *Food and Nutrition in the African Rain Forest*,
UNESCO/MAB, Paris, 92-4

De Garine, I. and Koppert G. (1988) Coping with seasonal fluctuations in
food supply among savanna populations: the Massa and Mussey of
Chad and Cameroon, in I. De Garine and G.A. Harrison (eds.), *Coping
with Uncertainty in Food Supply*, Clarendon Press, Oxford, 210-59

Drewnowski, A. and Greenwood M.R.C. (1983) Cream and sugar: human
preferences for high-fat foods, *Physiology of Behavior*, 30: 629-33

Dufour, D. (1987) Insects as food: a case study from the Northwest
Amazon, *American Anthropologist*, 89: 383-97

Dufour, D. (1992) Nutritional ecology in the tropical rain forests of
Amazonia, *American Journal of Human Biology*, 4: 197-207

Etkin, N.L. (1986) Multidisciplinary perspective in the interpretation of
plants used in indigenous medicine and diet, in N.L. Etkin (ed.), *Plants
in Indigenous Medicine and Diet*, Gordon and Breach Science Publishers
(Redgrave), New York, 2-30

Etkin, N.L. (1993) Anthropological methods in ethnopharmacology,
Journal of Ethnopharmacology, 38: 93-104

Etkin, N.L. and P. Ross (1991) Recasting malaria, medicine, and meals: A
perspective on disease adaptation, in L. Romanucci-Ross, D.E.
Moerman, and L.R. Tancredi (eds.), *The Anthropology of Medicine* (2nd
edn.), Praeger, New York, 230-58

Ferro-Luzzi, G.E. (1980) Food avoidances during the puerperium and
lactation in Tamilnadu, in J.R.K. Robson (ed.), *Food, Ecology, and Culture*,
Gordon and Breach, New York, 109-18

Fleuret, A. (1979) Methods for evaluation of the rôle of fruits and wild
greens in Shambaa diet: A case study, *Medical Anthropology*, 3: 249-69

Fleuret, A. (1986) Dietary and therapeutic used of fruit in three Taita
communities, in N.L. Etkin (ed.), *Plants in Indigenous Medicine and Diet*,
Gordon and Breach Science Publishers (Redgrave), New York, 151-70

Frisancho, A.R. (1979) *Human Adaptation*, Mosby, St Louis

Galef, B.G. (1988) Communication of information concerning distant diets
in a social central-place foraging species: *Rattus norvegicus*, in T. Zentall
and B.C. Galef (eds.), *Social Learning: A Comparative Approach*, Lawrence
Erlbaum, Hillsdale, N.J., 119-40

Glantz, M.H., (ed.) (1986) *Drought and Hunger in Africa*, Cambridge
University Press

Grivetti, L.E., Frentzel, C.J., Ginsberg, K.E., Howell, K.L. and Ogle, B.M.
(1987) Bush foods and edible weeds of agriculture: Perspectives on
dietary use of wild plants in Africa, their rôle in maintaining human
nutritional status and implications for agricultural development, in R.
Akhtar (ed.), *Health and Disease in Tropical Africa*, Harwood Publishers,
Chur, 51-81

Hames, R. (1992) Time allocation, in E.A. Smith and B. Winterhalder
(eds.), *Evolutionary Ecology and Human Behavior*, Aldine de Gruyter, New
York, 203-36

Hanson, A. and McMillan, D.E. (eds.) (1986) *Food in Africa*, Lynne Rienner, Boulder

Helman, C.G. (1990) *Culture, Health and Illness*, Wright, London

Hitchcock, R.K. (1989) Settlement, seasonality and subsistence stress among the Tyus of northern Botswana, in R. Huss-Ashmore, J. Curry and R. Hitchcock (eds.), *Coping with Seasonal Constraints*, MASCA, University of Pennsylvania, PA, 64-85

Hitchcock, R.K., Ebert, J.I. and Morgan, R.G. (1989) Drought, drought relief, and dependency among the Basarwa of Botswana, in R. Huss-Ashmore and S.H. Katz (eds.), *African Food Systems in Crisis, Part One: Microperspectives*, Gordon and Breach, New York, 303-36

Huss-Ashmore, R. and Katz, S.H. (eds.) (1989) *African food systems in crisis, Part One: Microperspectives*, Gordon and Breach, New York

Huss-Ashmore, R. and Glantz, M. (1993) Intra-household variation in diets of Swazi women and children, *American Journal of Physical Anthropology*, Supplement 16: 112 (abstract)

Huss-Ashmore, R. and Johnston, S.L. (1994) Wild plants as cultural adaptations to food stress, in N.L. Etkin (ed.), *Eating on the Wild Side*, University of Arizona Press, Tucson, 62-82

Irvine, F.R. (1952) Supplementary and emergency food plants of West Africa, *Economic Botany*, 6: 23-40

Iwu, M.M. (1986) Empirical investigations of dietary plants used in Igbo ethnomedicine, in N.L. Etkin (ed.), *Plants in Indigenous Medicine and Diet*, Gordon and Breach Science Publishers (Redgrave), New York, 131-50

Jackson, F.L.C. (1991) Secondary compounds in plants (allelochemicals) as promoters of human biological diversity, *Annual Reviews of Anthropology*, 20: 505-46

Jerome, N.W., Pelto, G.H. and Kandel R.F. (1980) An ecological approach to nutritional anthropology, in N.W. Jerome, R.F. Kandel and G.H. Pelto (eds.), *Nutritional Anthropology*, Redgrave, Pleasantville, N.Y., 13-46

Johns, T. (1986) Detoxification function of geophagy and domestication of the potato, *Journal of Chemical Ecology*, 12: 635-46

Johns, T. (1990) *With Bitter Herbs They Shall Eat It*, University of Arizona Press, Tucson

Johns, T. and Keen S.L. (1986) Taste evaluation of potato glycoalkaloids by the Aymara: a case study in human chemical ecology, *Human Ecology*, 14: 437-52

Johns, T. and Kubo (1988) A survey of traditional methods employed for the detoxification of plant foods, *Journal of Ethnobiology*, 8: 81-129

Jones, V.H. (1965) The bark of the bittersweet vine as an emergency food among the Indians of the western Great Lakes Region, *The Michigan Archaeologist*, 11: 170-80

Kaplan, H and Hill, K. (1992) The evolutionary ecology of food acquisition, in E.A. Smith and B. Winterhalder (eds.), *Evolutionary Ecology and Human Behavior*, Aldine de Gruyter, New York, 167-202

Katz, S.H. (1987) Food and biocultural evolution: A model for the investigation of modern nutritional problems, in F.E. Johnston (ed.), *Nutritional Anthropology*, Alan R. Liss, New York, 41-63

Keith, M. and Armelagos, G.J. (1983) Naturally occurring dietary and antibiotics and human health, in L. Romanucci-Ross, D.E. Moerman, and L.R. Tancredi (eds.), *The Anthropology of Medicine*, Bergen and Garvey, South Hadley, MA, 221-30

Kindscher, K. (1987) *Edible Wild Plants of the Prairie: An Ethnobotanical Guide*, University Press of Kansas, Lawrence

Krondl, M. and Lau, D. (1982) Social determinants in human food selection, in L.M. Barker (ed.), *The Psychobiology of Human Food Selection*, AVI Publishing Co., Westport, CT, 139-51

Kuhnlein, H.V. and Turner, M.J. (1991) *Traditional Plant Foods of Canadian Indigenous Peoples: Nutrition, Botany and Use*, Gordon and Breach Science Publishers, Philadelphia

Laferriere, J.E. (1992) Cultural and environmental response to drought among the Mountain Pima, *Ecology of Food and Nutrition*, 28: 1-9

Levitt, D. (1981) *Plants and people: Aboriginal uses of plants on Groote Eylandt*, Australian Institute of Aboriginal Studies, Canberra

Little, M. and Haas, J. (1989) *Human Population Biology*, Oxford University Press, New York

Little, M.A., Leslie, P.W. and Campbell, K.L. (1992) Energy reserves and parity of nomadic and settled Turkana women, *American Journal of Human Biology*, 4: 729-38

Logan, M.H. (1972) Humoral folk medicine: a potential aid in controlling pellagra in Mexico, *Ethnomedizin*, 4: 397-410

Malla, S.B., Rajbhandari, S.B., Shrestha, T.B., Adhikari, P.M., Adhikari, S.R. (eds.) (1982) *Wild Edible Plants of Nepal*, Department of Medicinal Plants, Kathmandu

May, J.M. (1961) *The Ecology of Malnutrition in the Far and Near East*, Hafner Publishing Co., New York

May, J.M. and McLellan, D.L. (1970) *The Ecology of Malnutrition in Eastern Africa and Four Countries of Western Africa*, Hafner Publishing Co., New York

McKay, D.A. (1980) Food, illness, and folk medicine: insights from Ulu Trengganu, West Malaysia, in J.R.K. Robson (ed.), *Food, Ecology and Culture*, Gordon and Breach, New York, 61-6

Miller, J. and Huss-Ashmore, R. (1989) Do reproductive patterns affect maternal nutritional status? An analysis of maternal depletion in Lesotho, *American Journal of Human Biology*, 1: 409-19

Nabhan, G.P. (1989) *Enduring Seeds: Native American Agriculture and Wild Plant Conservation*, North Point Press, San Francisco

National Research Council (1989) *Lost Crops of the Incas: Little-known Plants of the Andes with Promise for Worldwide Cultivation*, Report of an Ad Hoc Panel of the Advisory Committee on Technology Innovation, Board on Science and Technology for International Development, National Academy Press, Washington, D.C.

Ogbu, J.O. (1973) Seasonal hunger in tropical Africa as a cultural phenomenon: The Onicha Ibo of Nigeria and Chakaka Poka of Malawi examples, *Africa*, 43: 317-332

Pagezy, H. (1990) Feeding the primiparous mother among the Ntomba of Zaire, in *Food and Nutrition in the African Rain Forest*, C.M. Hladik, S. Bahuchet, and I. de Garine (eds.), UNESCO/MAB, Paris, 89-91

Pyke, G.H. (1984) Optimal foraging theory: a critical review, *Annual Review of Ecology and Systematics*, 15: 523-75

Pyke, I.L. and Winterbauer, N.L. (1993) Anthropometric indicators of seasonal and annual variation in health and nutritional status in nomadic Turkana pastoralists, *American Journal of Physical Anthropology*, Supplement 16: 158-9

Quin, P.J. (1959) *Food and Feeding Habits of the Pedi, with Special Reference to Identification, Classification, Preparation and Nutritive Value of the Respective Foods*, Witwatersrand University Press, Johannesburg

Rahmato, D. (1991) *Famine and Survival Strategies*, Nordiska Afrika Institutet, Uppsala

Read, B.E. (1977) *Famine Foods Listed in the Chiu Huang Pen Ts'ao Giving their Identity, Nutritional Values and Notes on their Preparation* (Reprint of 1946 publication), Southern Materia Medica Center, Inc., Taipei

Regmi, P.P. (1982) *An Introduction to Nepalese Food Plants*, Royal Nepal Academy, Kathmandu

Riley, B.W. and Brokensha, D. (1988) *The Mbeere of Kenya, Volume I: Changing Rural Ecology*, Institute for Development Anthropology, University Press of America, Lanham, Maryland

Robson, J.R.K. (ed.) (1981) *Famine: Its Causes, Effects and Management*, Gordon and Breach, New York

Rozin, E. (1982) The structure of cuisine, in L.M. Barker (ed.), *The Psychobiology of Human Food Selection*, AVI Publishing Co. Westport, CT, 189-204

Rozin, P.N. (1982) Human food selection: the interaction of biology, culture, and individual experience, in *The Psychobiology of Human Food Selection*, L.M. Barker (ed.), AVI Publishing Co., Westport, CT, 225-53

Rozin, P.N. (1990) Acquisition of stable food preferences, *Nutrition Reviews*, 48: 106-113

Rozin, P.N. and Schulkin J. (1990) Food selection, in E.M. Stricker (ed.), *Handbook of Behavioral Neurobiology*, Plenum Press, New York, 297-328

Scudder, T. (1971) *Gathering Among African Woodland Savanna Cultivators, a Case Study: The Gwembe Tonga*, University of Zambia Institute Studies, Lusaka

Singh, H.B. and Arora, R.K. (1978) *Wild Edible Plants of India*, Indian Council of Agricultural Research, New Delhi

Smith, E.A. (1983) Anthropological applications of optimal foraging theory: a critical review, *Current Anthropology*, 24: 625-51

Solbrig, O.T. and Orians, G.H. (1977) The adaptive characteristics of desert plants, *American Scientist*, 65: 412-21

Stahl, A.B. (1984) Hominid dietary selection before fire, *Current Anthropology*, 24: 151-68

Steegman, A.T. (1983) Boreal forest hazards and adaptations: The past, in A.T. Steegman (ed.), *Boreal Forest Adaptations: The Northern Algonkians*, Plenum Press, New York, 243-67

Steward, J.H. (1938) *Basin-Plateau Aboriginal Sociopolitical Groups*, Bureau of American Ethnology Bulletin, United States Government Printing Office, Washington, D.C., 120

Sukkakry-Stolba, S. (1989) Indigenous institutions and adaptation to famine: The case of the Western Sudan, in R. Huss-Ashmore and S.H. Katz (eds.), *African Food Systems in Crisis, Part One: Microperspectives*, Gordon and Breach, New York, 281-94

Watts, M. (1983) *Silent Violence*, University of California Press, Berkeley

Wilson, C.S. (1980) Food taboos of childbirth: the Malay example, in J.R.K. Rubstone (ed.), *Food Ecology and Culture*, Gordon and Breach, New York, 67-74

8. THREE CENTURIES OF CHANGING EUROPEAN TASTES FOR THE POTATO

Ellen Messer

In 1992 two cookbooks devoted exclusively to potatoes, Lydie Marshall's *A Passion for Potatoes* and Lindsey Bareham's *In Praise of the Potato*, published hundreds of recipes – many of them from Europe – for potato appetizers, soups, salads, main courses, and even desserts. They testified how the ever adaptable tuber, *Solanum tuberosum*, over several centuries, had captured the tastes of European consumers, and helped shape their cuisines. In the years surrounding 1992, quincentennary symposia marking Columbus' 1492 encounter with New World peoples and products, including the potato, presented plant scientists, anthropologists, and historians with opportunities to assess the impacts of five-hundred years of potato 'exchange' that involved changing European tastes for the potato (Viola and Margolis, 1991). These mostly ecological accounts recalled in particular the significance of the potato in Irish history, especially the Great Hunger of 1845-1847. In connection with the sesquicentennial of this series of crop failures, they retraced the ecological and political steps leading up to the calamitous famine (Kinealy, 1994). However, curiously few probed in comparable detail the development of Irish or other European tastes for potatoes.

Sidney Mintz, in an essay entitled 'Food and its relationship to power' (Mintz, 1996), suggests that to understand the acceptance of new foods, changing tastes, and the mechanisms by which new dietary components and patterns become established, anthropologists (or others) need to answer not one but two sets of questions. First, under what circumstances do people accept new foods and change food habits? Second, having accommodated new foods for reasons not necessarily of their own choosing, how do people create 'new consumption situations endowed with new meanings they themselves have engineered?' (1996: 17).

To answer these questions, he suggests a dual outsider-insider perspective. Outsider dimensions include the political-economic, environmental, commercial, and biological forces beyond any individual's, household's, or cultural community's control. Most political-economic treatments of the potato in Europe, and in Ireland in particular, tend toward 'outsider' dimensions, focusing either on demographic imperatives or political-economic exploitation and injustice (e.g., Ross, 1986).

By contrast, insider dimensions ponder the decisions that people make regarding dietary choices and structures. They consider the determinants of food intake, dietary structure and content, and describe sensory, economic, prestige, and symbolic factors influencing tastes and nutritional habits, especially those in the process of change (Messer, 1984). They also emphasise ways particular foods are integrated into everyday life and cultural meanings.

Mintz furthermore suggests that major changes in consumption habits are usually brought on by major disruptions in ordinary routines. To change food preferences and dietary structures there probably need to be not only the right ecological and political conditions but also some major social rupture that creates an opening for a new food or nutrition pattern and a reason for abandoning the old. In his examples, war constitutes a major category of social upheaval that creates contexts characterised by new food and nutrition needs as well as new opportunities (Mintz, 1996). Other disjunctures providing occasions for dietary change include migration, involving population movements from one to another country, from rural to urban areas within a single country, or a restructuring of population on existing land as a result of agricultural reform or industrial change (see discussion of immigration and change in food preferences in chapter 14, this volume).

In addition, culinary dimensions or nutritional-health factors are sometimes important in shaping where, when, and how a new product is integrated into the cultural diet and cosmology. Culinary qualities are also linked to biological characteristics of food species, such as particular tastes and cooking characteristics of distinctive varieties, about which there may be more or less historical information.

Evolving tastes for the potato in Europe over three hundred years involved 'outsider' dimensions such as potato biology, ecology, and agronomy; as well as economic necessity and political promotion or coercion. Against this background, 'insider' frameworks fit the potato into European diets as a humble famine or staple food of the lower classes; a prestigious vegetable food of élites; or as an ingredient of national dishes or cuisines that set one potato-eating European population apart from another. Historic disjunctures included agricultural reforms, new trade rules, and demographic changes associated with the industrial revolution and agricultural enclosures. All helped provoke or accelerate the pace of dietary change among resistant European populations.

Outsider Perspectives

In nutritional and agricultural terms, the potato, *Solanum tuberosum*, with hundreds of locally adapted varieties, produces more calories and protein per unit area and labour than any other major grain or root crop. Eaten in quantity, it provides adequate calories, good quality protein, and also furnishes protective quantities of vitamin C, a micronutrient that was sometimes scarce in the diets of marginal peasants and industrial workers of early modern Europe. Properly stored and completely cooked, the potato is non-toxic, tasty, and filling; it offers nutritious food, easily prepared by simple boiling or baking, and is good to eat, even alone with salt and without more costly condiments.

The potato is also extremely adaptable to climate and other environmental extremes. It responds favourably to intensive gardening but some varieties yield well with minimal care or chemicals. Quick yields (some varieties set tubers after only sixty days) make the potato an unrivalled famine food in areas where previous grain crops have fallen short, and also an important seasonal ('hunger') crop where intercropped with cereals. It also can be stored underground and retrieved as needed; an advantage in wartime over grain stocks, which can be burned or seized. But it cannot be stored over multiple years or shipped easily – a disadvantage in trade or times of famine.

Political-economic circumstances magnified the biological advantages. In rural areas, agricultural reforms were making land increasingly scarce for small farmers who had relied on common lands for grazing and cropping. In urban zones, industrial developments were giving rise to burgeoning populations who needed a cheap food staple. Although bread, followed by gruels, were the familiar and preferred staple foods, workers increasingly could not afford to eat grain, only potatoes.

Militating against quick acceptance of the potato, however, were other biological and cultural factors. The earliest introduced potato varieties faced a biological-ecological barrier: they did not yield well in the long summer days of temperate Europe. Drawings reveal these were short-day *andigena* rather than long-day *tuberosum* types; so most would not have set tubers until the shorter, but colder autumn days. Selection for suitable varieties took at least a hundred years. Europeans were also utterly unfamiliar with roots or tubers as a staple crop. Roots and tubers were at this time, at most, winter vegetables not staple foods, and they were reproduced from seeds, not eyes or cuttings. Furthermore, unlike maize, potatoes could not be easily made into bread. European botanists and physicians, moreover, classified the potato as 'windy' and indigestible, a food fit only for peasants or animals. These characteristics in part explain why European adoption was selective and took close to three hundred years for the potato to be accepted throughout Europe.

Insider Perspectives

Sixteenth-century Spanish explorers who first encountered the potato in South America compared the unfamiliar tuber in taste to truffles, that also grew underground. They observed hundreds of varieties, and also freeze-dried potatoes, but neither multiple varieties nor processing techniques accompanied potatoes to Europe. The first specimens probably reached Spain circa 1570. From there, an important source of diffusion and information were herbalists, such as Gerard, who described, depicted and named the new tuber. Regrettably, by the doctrine of signatures' principle of similarity (like causes like), they likened potatoes to the withered extremities of lepers; also to sexual parts, for which the potato acquired repellant names such as 'Eve's apple' or 'earth's testicles'. Such an unwholesome reputation contributed to avoidance of potatoes in Burgundy, and for some time later in France, Germany, and Russia but not in the British Isles.

Ireland and England

In England and Ireland, there were probably separate potato introductions circa 1590 (although probably not from Sir Francis Drake or the Spanish Armada, as claimed in local folklore), and potatoes were (erroneously, but patriotically) labelled to be from 'Virginia' (a

British colony), then 'Irish' and finally 'white'. Ireland, where warm days extended into the autumn, had the advantage that short-day potato varieties yielded adequately. As farmers selected for later-yielding, disease-resistant and tasty varieties, the potato entered Irish diets in four stages:

1. as supplementary food and defence against famine (1590-1675);
2. as winter food for the poor, based on its superior yields and minimal processing costs relative to grains; early-sown varieties predominant (1675-1750);
3. as staple food of small farmers over most of the year and an important food in the diet of all classes; the so-called 'golden age' of the potato culture when such varieties as 'black' and 'apple' with superior taste and keeping qualities, and later the less durable 'cup' were widely grown (1750-1810); and
4. as barely edible food of last resort; in decline toward famine, people relied on the watery, late-sown and late-yielding 'lumper' variety, considered scarcely adequate even for animal feed outside of Ireland (1810-1845) (Bourke, 1993).

As landlords made less land and time available for self-provisioning, potatoes were fit into an evolving 'conacre' custom or economy, which allowed landless peasants to rent small plots for eleven-month periods, in return for agricultural services to the landlord. Peasants managed to feed themselves on such miniscule holdings by setting up raised 'lazy' beds that yielded abundantly in the few months between the harvest of the previous and the sowing of the subsequent grain crops. They provided most of the following year's subsistence for the poorest peasants and a nutritional interval in the diets of slightly more fortunate peasants who also had access to some grains and animal foods. In addition to being filling and tasty for humans, potatoes and skins could be fed to livestock, which provided nourishment and income, even for humble tenant farmers. The better-off smallholders also ate some oatmeal, wheat bread, milk, and pork. These accommodations to the political economy of Irish grain production and trade, which left land mostly in the hands of absent British landlords, were dimensions of 'internal' response to 'external' conditions that shaped acceptance of potatoes as a major food. Acceptance and integration of the potato was also facilitated over the seventeenth and eighteenth century by the availability of multiple varieties, each more or less preferred for certain dishes, or relegated to animals. Until the tastier and more durable varieties such as 'black' and 'apple' were undermined by disease, the potato happily provided a flexible and diverse culinary ingredient, around which the Irish constructed an entire national cuisine which endures in Irish cooking, literature, and culture today.

By the eighteenth century multiple sturdy potato varieties with different flavours provided the ingredients for a varied cuisine that in innovative ways combined potatoes as a dominant ingredient with more expensive but more customary grains, fats, meats. Potatoes (also called 'murphies' or 'praties'), in addition to being eaten boiled, baked, or roasted in or out of their skins, alone or with a dip of milk or salted fish, developed as the principal ingredient in 'colcannon' (boiled mashed potatoes with cabbage and leeks), which was festival fare for Hallowe'en and All Souls/All Saint's Day, and 'champ' (mashed potatoes with onions and milk), that celebrated the harvest of new potatoes. Additionally, both these dishes were celebrated with song and dance. Other typical potato preparations included 'boxty' (mashed potatoes with flour) bread or pancakes; apple potato cake or 'fadge' and numerous stews, soups, puffs, and farls that came to define Irish cuisine before and after the famine. Possibly selection for floury varieties contributed to successful elaboration of some of these dishes (Mahon, 1991), although we have almost no guidance on varieties from the sources. Folkloric and culinary sources suggest that such culinary developments did not occur overnight but some two centuries elapsed between the introduction of potatoes and their thorough integration into Irish cuisine (Mahon, 1991). In 1845, the first year of the famine, the potato crop occupied some two million acres and there was anticipated a 13.6 million ton harvest, of which slightly less than half would have gone to humans, who as adults consumed six to fourteen pounds of potatoes per day.

Outside rural areas, potatoes also provided a cheap food source for industrial workers. Salaman (1949), Hobhouse (1986), and McNeill (1974) all credit potatoes with having allowed the rapid rise of population associated with the Industrial Revolution and urbanization in England and later in Europe, a socioeconomic-demographic finding that rather negatively impressed Malthus (1798), who predicted calamity, should the potato crop fail, and Adam Smith (1776) who more positively credited potato with increasing the wealth of nations (and the beauty of Irish women!). The potato's main disadvantage, according to Smith, was that unlike less highly productive grains, it could not be stored from year to year. With the exception of Salaman (1949), who was originally a potato scientist, none of these political-economic sources discusses explicitly that different varieties of potatoes have different culinary or taste qualities, and are more or less suitable for particular geographic zones, or more or less vulnerable to particular pests. Malthus, however, in his gloomy demographic prognosis, recognised the susceptibility of the potato species to diseases, including viruses and fungi, that in Ireland by the early nineteenth century brought the 'golden age' of potatoes (1750-1810), with its superior and tastier but more vulnerable varieties, to a close.

The European Mainland

Negative folklore notwithstanding, potatoes by 1650 were mentioned as a field crop of Flanders, by 1697 had spread northward to Zeeland, by 1731 to Utrecht, by 1746 to Overijseel, and by 1765 to Friesland. They were adopted as a field crop and anti-famine food of high altitude areas and spread rapidly especially after the hard winter of 1740 that damaged grain crops. By 1794 they had been accepted as an element of the Dutch national dish, a hot pot of root vegetables (Davidson, 1992). Culinary historians generally interpret this to have been a very slow process (e.g., Davidson, 1992), but the timing roughly parallels that of the Irish, who are usually interpreted to have been earlier and less resistant adopters. The transition from adoption to enjoyment of the taste is probably a function of habituation and cultural coding. Throughout Europe people learned to enjoy the potato by making it their own, i.e., by combining it with more typical foods and flavourings, sometimes into typical dishes.

Acceptance was somewhat more retarded in Germany, where potatoes continued to be resisted by farmers, but where too, by the end of the eighteenth century, they had become a field crop with especially large production after famine and war years. Farmers were ordered to grow potatoes as a hedge against famine, a more highly productive crop, and also as a protective measure in wartime, since potatoes, if stored in the ground, could not be burned. Potato adoption was also tied to the never-ending wars in Germany, where they quickly changed the art of provisioning (McNeill, 1974); the War of the Bavarian Succession (1778-1779), was even nicknamed the *Kartoffelkrieg* ('potato war') because it lasted only as long as there were potatoes to feed the soldiers, who, living off the land, dug them from the fields as they ravaged the countryside.

This German war also unintentionally influenced the popularisation of potatoes in France because Parmentier, a French pharmacist who had been a prisoner of war in Germany and fed on potatoes, promoted them upon his return home. He grew potatoes and convinced Marie Antoinette to wear potato flowers in her hair and Louis

XV to wear them as boutaniers. Parmentier tried to popularise potato as a flour extender. However, widespread potato consumption in France still had to wait another century because potato starch added to wheat flour produced an unacceptably soggy bread that was too moist to sop up soup at a time when bread and soup were French dietary staples (Wheaton, 1983). Curiously, not until the next century do French cooks seem to have had access to the most flavourful varieties or to have mastered the French art of meshing potatoes with the flavours of other foods (Wheaton, 1983). Although a 1600 natural history report by De Serre (cited in Wheaton, 1983) had compared the potato's taste favourably to truffles (he even called it 'cartoufle', like, or perhaps copying, the Spanish), in the eighteenth century French opinion makers still despised potatoes as insipid and causing flatulence. Widespread utilisation of the whole potato in soup, fries, or other forms did not occur until the following century.

By that time the poorest class of peasant cultivators probably were forced by economic circumstances to eat potatoes when they could not afford bread, whereas wealthier classes had adopted potatoes as a luxury vegetable; double-fried (or 'souffléed') potatoes are apocryphally linked to Louis XVI (1830). Suitable varieties would have been important in bringing about such culinary changes but information is scant. Perhaps the most penetrating evidence for still divided French judgments on potato is Millet's famous painting, *The Potato Planters* (1861) that raised a storm of critical indignation against ennobling such a 'vulgar' subject (Murphy, 1984). Millet's beautiful and monumental treatment of the humble planters testifies that by the 1860s potatoes were well-known peasant crops and food in France. Meanwhile, some, but not all, members of high society, placed high value on potatoes and their cultivators for being so close to nature (see van Tilbourgh, 1993).

By the middle eighteenth through nineteenth centuries, potatoes finally spread across Central and Eastern Europe into Russia. Peter the Great, at the end of the seventeenth century, was reported to have sent a sack of potatoes home, where their production was promoted first by the Free Economic Society and a century later by government land grants. But as late as 1840 'Old Believers' continued to reject potatoes as 'Devil's apples' or 'forbidden fruits of Eden' that were unsuitable for human consumption. When in that year the government finally ordered peasant farmers to grow potatoes on common lands, the peasants responded with 'potato riots' that lasted until 1843 when the coercive policy ceased. Over the next half century, however, farmers voluntarily adopted potatoes as a garden vegetable and then as a field crop, encouraged by the potato's obvious superiority to most grain crops and other tubers. They appear in many variations in Russian cookbooks by the end of the century (Toomre, 1992); by the Russian civil wars and World Wars of the early twentieth century they were clearly Russia's 'second bread'.

Power, Political-Economy and Meaning

By the middle of the nineteenth century potatoes were providing cheap food for the increasing populations all over Europe. It had taken almost three centuries in some places to overcome superstitions that potatoes were poisonous, tasteless, hard-to-digest, and aphrodisiac; or aversions to potato as pig food, famine-food, or food for the poor. Over this time, European potato varieties had evolved that were better adapted to the longer-day conditions of temperate Europe and demonstrably more highly productive than grain crops in the same environments. Gardeners and farmers had been able to demonstrate their superior productivity and their harmlessness. Land-poor peasants, facing production constraints and rising consumer prices for grains, had been able to fit the potato into crop rotations and new productive niches where nothing else guaranteed subsistence. And industrialists and potentates found potatoes met the need of growing urban populations for a low-cost staple food.

Once adopted, each European culture constructed its own distinctive potato cuisine and tastes around particular potato varieties and dishes. The tuber species offered many varieties with multiple possibilities, some better than others for boiling, baking, mashing, or frying. Suitable varieties were turned into mashed potato puddings, breads or pancakes by the Irish and English, soufflés or gratins by the French, gnocchi by Italians, dumplings by eastern Europeans, or stews, soups or salads by Dutch and Germans. Social and cultural value on consuming bread, as in France, worked against the adoption of a staple food such as potato. In England and Ireland, diets that already included various grains and gruels depending on season and social status proved more adaptable in adopting the potato. This situation probably also characterised areas of the Low Countries, Central and Eastern Europe that adopted and adapted potato as a co-staple food, sometimes along with maize, another New World crop.

Most of the early varieties, derived from original *andigena* introductions, were wiped out by late blight, but they were replaced by the blight-resistant and superior European *tuberosum* varieties including Bintje (Netherlands, 1910), King Edward (U.K., 1902) and others that are still specified in contemporary recipes for baked, fried, or other potato dishes (Jellis and Richardson, 1987). Although mass potato production for the post-Second World War preference of standardised fries and snacks has over the years selected for more insipid spuds, a countervailing demand has arisen for old-fashioned (now gourmet) potatoes, such as the French La Ratte or 'la Reine,' a dense, golden-fleshed variety boasting 'a flavour that hints richly of hazelnuts and chestnuts' (Fabricant, 1996). Such culinary fare returns the potato eater to late sixteenth and early seventeenth century descriptions of early European potato varieties. It also raises once again the issues of culinary fashions and revolutions in tastes, or the circumstances which provoke changes in food habits.

Revolutions in Politics and Taste

Wars were a contributing factor to the adoption of the potato in Europe, most explicitly in Germany, but also in other cases, such as Ireland; and later in Eastern Europe and Russia, where warfare raised the need for more and safer food that could be provided by underground crops. Acceptance of potatoes in early modern Europe was also part of other major social and political-economic revolutions, including the Industrial Revolution; the scientific agricultural revolution; and capitalist (mercantilist) trade revolutions, all of which were instrumental in bringing about transformations in European food tastes over a two to three hundred year period. These characteristics in part explain why it took close to three hundred years for the potato to be accepted throughout Europe.

In early modern Europe, these revolutions were settings where, to paraphrase Mintz (1996: 28), outside political economic processes imposed many of the conditions within which inside meanings took shape. In the case of the potato, intrinsic nutritional value and agricultural properties were of great significance, but so was the dearth of other foods. Potatoes were introduced into social circumstances where populations were already in upheaval, where food habits were already or would soon be in a process of change. The adoption of potato in these historical cases proves to have been not so much a departure from traditional foods and stable dietary patterns as a new element that allowed people to find a new pattern of subsistence where the old was no longer viable. In much the same fashion, tea and white bread replaced the potato in Irish and British urban diets after the famine.

Recent expansions of potato-eating in Africa and Asia are linked to other food and social revolutions, including the agricultural

'Green Revolution' (and more recently the biotechnology revolution) in the developing world. Since 1972 activities of the International Potato Center have encouraged rapid increase in potato production and consumption in Asia, Africa, and Latin America. Tastes for potatoes are also being spread via the food industry; in particular the industrialised food processing and multinational agribusinesses and restaurant businesses bring potato fries, chips, and snacks in standard fast food formats to peoples all over the world. Although the acceptance of potato in these fatty fast food forms are the products of 'outsider' commercial and political interests, for people newly arrived in urban areas from many different cultures, acceptance has been internally structured to be snacks by people on the run without time to eat formal meals or sociable foods.

Beyond these mostly urban contexts, potatoes in developing countries, as had been the case historically in Europe, have been adopted to fit high altitude agricultural niches where no other major staple food grows; as a protective food against famine at lower altitudes, and as a co-staple with grains and legumes where these other crops are in short supply (Furer-Haimendorf, 1964; C.I.P., 1984). In Asia and Africa as in historical Europe, the potato serves as a staple food of the poor or a higher status vegetable, and has experienced its greatest growth as a seasonal food and cash intercrop with more accustomed cereal grains (Van der Zaag, 1984). In contrast to Europe, though, guarding against dangerous overdependence on the potato and potential potato famines are very different traditions and conditions of land tenure; more diverse seeding materials; and international agricultural efforts that struggle against omnipresent spectres of blight (C.I.P., 1984).

In most places diversified tastes for multiple food staples offer both the wealthy and the poor many more food options.

Conclusion

Three centuries of changing European tastes for the potato illustrate that adoption and enjoyment of a new food cannot occur until the item is available. It may then take some time for 'tastes' to develop. Tastes develop either out of economic necessity (the potato is the only item that is available or affordable) or because an item becomes truly desirable, having been integrated via additional cultural coding into the familiar cuisine (the potato is prepared and flavoured into typical, even ritual dishes). Militating against easy acceptance are unpleasant, poisonous or apparently unhealthful characteristics; also the association of an item with disadvantage. The piece that is missing in this history is more reliable information on taste. There is regrettably little specific information in most histories on what constituted desirable taste characteristics or tasty varieties. We know that the Irish 'lumper' variety was considered to be untasty, in contrast to 'black' or 'cup'. It was described as watery, insipid, barely edible for humans and later-yielding and less durable. Food folklore extolls the earlier varieties, that were undermined by disease. We can only surmise that they were less insipid and that they tasted more like the denser, more flavourful varieties described earlier and later (e.g., La Ratte). Preferences for certain varieties most likely were associated with the types and amounts of elaboration; in the case of the Irish, different potatoes were preferred for boiling, colcannon, or fries, but again, there is not a great deal of ready information. Significantly, the European potatoes, in contrast to Andean potatoes, also appear to have been benign, not bitter, so that no taste selection was involved to avoid unpleasant or toxic taste qualities.

In the end, we return to the finding that political-economic factors had a great deal of influence on the development of tastes for potato, but intrinsic biological characteristics of the potato, and cultural factors in cuisine, were also instrumental in the adoption and integration of potato into European cuisines.

References

Bareham, L. (1992) *In Praise of the Potato*, Overlook Press, Woodstock, New York

Bourke, A. (1993) *'The Visitation of God?' The Potato and the Great Irish Famine*, The Lilliput Press, Dublin

C.I.P. (International Potato Centre) (1984) *Potatoes for the Developing World: A Collaborative Experience*, C.I.P., Lima

Davidson, A. (1992) The Europeans' wary encounter with tomatoes, potatoes and other New World foods, in N. Foster and L.S. Cordell (eds.) *Chillies to Chocolate: Food the Americas Gave the World*, University of Arizona, Phoenix

Fabricant, F. (1996) French revolution in potatoes comes to America, *New York Times*, 25 September 1996, C6

Furer-Haimendorf, C. von (1964) *The Sherpas of Nepal: Buddhist Highlanders*, John Murray, London

Hobhouse, H. (1986) *Seeds of Change: Five Plants that Transformed the World,* Harper & Row, New York

Jellis, G.J. and Richardson, D.E. (1987) The development of potato varieties in Europe, in G.J. Jellis and D.E. Richardson (eds.) *The Production of New Potato Varieties: Technological Advances,* Cambridge University Press

Kinealy, C. (1994) *The Great Calamity: the Irish Famine 1845-52,* Roberts Rinehart, Boulder

Mahon, B. (1991) *The Land of Milk and Honey: the Story of Traditional Irish Food and Drink,* Poolbeg Press, Dublin

Malthus, T. (1798) *Essay on Population,* London

Marshall, L. (1992) *A Passion for Potatoes,* Harper Perennial, New York

McNeill, W.H. (1974) *The Shape of European History,* Oxford University Press, New York

Messer, E. (1984) Anthropological perspectives on diet, *Annual Review of Anthropology,* 13: 205-50

Mintz, S. (1996) *Tasting Food, Tasting Freedom,* Beacon Press, Boston

Murphy, A. (1984) *Millet,* Museum of Fine Arts, Boston

Ross, E. (1986) Potatoes, population and the Irish famine: the political economy of demographic change, in W.P. Handworker (ed.) *Culture and Reproduction,* Westview, Boulder, Colorado

Salaman, R.N. (1985) *The History and Social Influence of the Potato,* Cambridge (original publication 1949)

Smith, A. (1776) *An Inquiry into the Nature and Causes of the Wealth of Nations,* E. Cannon (ed.), London (1904-50 edition)

van Tilborgh, L. (1993) *The Potato Eaters by Vincent van Gogh,* Waanders, Zwolle

Toomre, J. (1992) *Classic Russian Cooking: Elena Molokhovets' A Gift to Young Housewives (1861-1975),* Indiana University Press, Bloomington

Van der Zaag, P. (1984) One potato, two potato, *Far Eastern Economic Review,* 23 August 1984: 64-6

Vincent, J. (1995) Conacre: a re-evaluation of Irish custom, in J. Schneider and R. Rapp (eds.) *Articulating Hidden Histories: Exploring the Influence of Eric Wolf,* University of California, Berkeley

Viola, H. and Margolis, C (eds.) (1991) *Seeds of Change: a Quincentennial Commemorative,* Smithsonian, Washington D.C.

Wheaton, B. (1983) *Savoring the Past: the French Kitchen and Tables from 1300 to 1789,* University of Pennsylvania Press, Philadelphia

9. THE PATHWAYS OF TASTE
THE WEST ANDALUCIAN CASE

*Isabel González Turmo** *

Introduction

Analysis of food preferences and taste can become an important key to the understanding of cultural differences over and above the simple description of what is observed. Food preferences involve hopes and compromises with reality that have an interesting relationship with social conditions and concepts of identity. By gathering both ethnographic and quantitative data on food habits and diet, information that is at the same time both broad and detailed can throw light on this relationship. This study is based on an example of such all-inclusive research. It concerns fieldwork carried out between 1987 and 1993 in the provinces of Seville, Cadiz and Huelva (Map 9.1). These provinces are in the most westerly part of Andalucia, a region of 87,267 square kilometres, which is divided between the broad depression of the Guadalquivir, extensive mountain ranges and more than 800 km of coastline, partly Atlantic and partly Mediterranean. The Guadalquivir river runs east to west and its basin occupies almost seventy percent of the territory under discussion.

This research began as part of a much larger project initiated by the French CNRS to study human food habits in marine and marsh ecosystems: the French Camargue, the mouth of the San Pedro river in Mexico and the mouth of the Guadalquivir in Andalucia.

* Translated by Helen Macbeth

Map 9.1 Map of Andalucia showing western villages studied

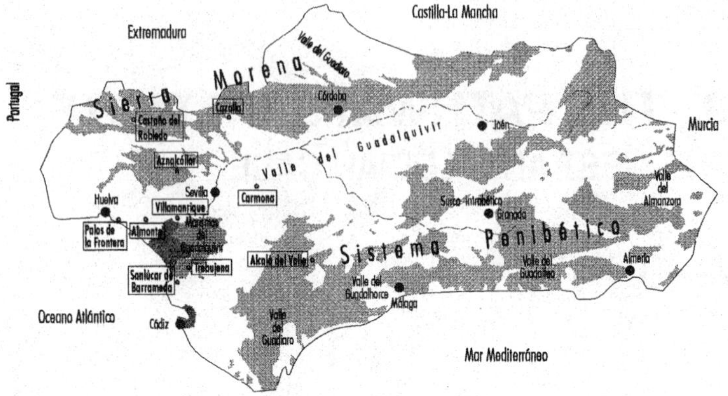

Geographic Setting and Population Samples

The marshlands of the Guadalquivir and the Doñana Reservation constitute a vast triangle of marshes and lands with sandy substrata called *cotos*. The huge marshy plain is crossed by the Guadalquivir which beyond Seville runs slowly. The intricate network of subsidiary streams that until recently furrowed this land has been much altered in recent decades. Nevertheless the plentiful water continues to be the principal source of wealth. This wealth and an interest in 'natural' ecosystems have motivated 'conservation' politics, which have set up the National Park of the Doñana (50,720 hectares) and the Natural Park of the Entorno de la Doñana (54,200 hectares) (Map 9.2).

This extensive and practically uninhabited territory is surrounded by densely populated urban and suburban centres. The choice of this region for the first phase of the research rested on three important factors which coincided in this area:

1. some food habits have been recently acquired because of new retailing networks;
2. some largely rural communes could be called traditionally Andalucian; and
3. there is still some use of wild foods, obtained through gathering, hunting, and river and coastal fishing.

Map 9.2 Map of National and Natural Parks of Doñana

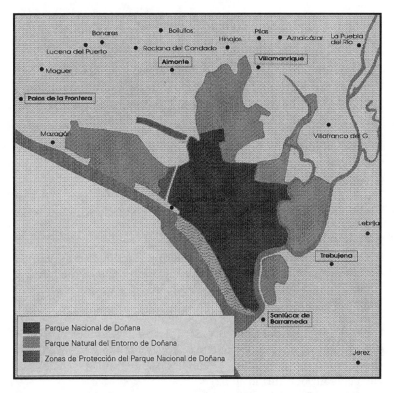

Parque Nacional de Doñana
Parque Natural del Entorno de Doñana
Zonas de Protección del Parque Nacional de Doñana

Source: Comisión Internacional de Expertos sobre el Desarrollo del Entorno de Doñana.
Dictamen sobre estrategias para el desarrollo sostenible de Doñana. Junta de Andalucía. 1992.

For the fieldwork in this area, four sample populations were chosen: Sanlucar de Barrameda and Trebujena in the province of Cadiz, Villamanrique in Seville, and Almonte in Huelva (Map 9.1). However, early results after two years of fieldwork showed that the people of the Doñana Reservation and the Marshlands of the Guadalquivir did not have distinctive food habits, but rather customs similar to those in the rural areas of most of southern Andalucia. It was even doubtful if there was anything significantly different about the hunting and gathering by the people from the marshlands as wild foods were also abundant in the hills. The study was therefore extended to include: Palos de la Frontera and Castaño del Robledo in Huelva, Aznalcollar, Cazalla de la Sierra and Carmona in Seville, and Alcala del Valle in Cadiz (Map 9.1). Villages were chosen which maximised the environmental contrasts between them, because the intention was to review the role of social and environmental factors in regard to food choices and habits.

Methods

Ethnographic information was gathered from interviewing the residents of these areas. The interviewing techniques were of three kinds: in-depth interviews, extensive interviews and specialist interviews, described below.

In-depth interviews

These were open and semistructured and aimed at domestic groups, including all family members. The topics covered were:

1. *Diet:* quantities, composition, preferences, continuity and change at home and in the workplace;
2. *Processing:* preparation and preservation of foods;
3. *Origin:* marketing, production, gathering, hunting and fishing;
4. *Attitudes:* taste, nutritional knowledge, dedication to the kitchen, table behaviour, commensality, invitations and festivities;
5. *Special conditions:* pregnancy, lactation, sickness, age.

For each of the above, differences by age, gender and socioeconomic status were considered. Complete interviews of three to seven days were carried out in eighty-three families, a minimum of eight in each village (González Turmo, 1992).

Extensive interviews

There were also briefer interviews, a minimum of twenty in each village, to quantify food intake.

Specialist interviews

These interviews were directed at individuals and groups involved in food production and related industries.

From these interviews a rich fund of information on food habits in this region has been obtained. The most relevant material on taste was gathered under the heading of diet, because not only was each family member asked about their individual preferences, but also the housewife was asked to discuss her specialities. These data were then compared with actual diet as shown in the food intake and shopping records. Also, individuals were asked about food desires and longings, and what changes they would make to diet and kitchen if they had plenty of money.

Results

It was noted that people in each village and even each district *(comarca)* stated preferences for those foods provided by their own environment, or those which were part of their culinary traditions: for example, fish on the coast, pork products where people had pigs, etc. This did not mean that the rest did not eat such items. In fact, no significant differences in food intake were shown by locality.

The influence of social status on taste was more significant. The few members of the rich élite exhibited tastes which could be described in accordance with their wealthy circumstances. They could eat anything they wished. Some, however, wanted to return to a cuisine considered 'traditional'. The middle classes and the *nouveaux riches*, on the other hand, were alike in their preferences: many desired more ham and more shellfish, both of which are considered symbols of luxury and economic power. Those in the villages of the interior would also have liked to have a better grade of fish. Finally, the lower classes were happy to eat exactly what they do eat. The fishermen like nothing better than fish and there is no dish more appreciated by a farmworker than a stew made of meat or pulses. Although for celebrations these too buy ham and shellfish, what is important for them is that there is no lack, *La abundancia!* Along the same lines, many members of these classes confessed that they generally did not like unfamiliar foods, but preferred those of everyday.

As far as seasonality was concerned the preferences expressed by the different social classes were on the whole not found to be dissimilar, but what they actually ate did show differences. There is a general preference for cold and light meals in summer. Over the last couple of decades these have been progressively replacing the traditional dishes, but that does not mean that everyone can afford them. In fact, many are unable to afford the spring produce or to augment their diet with greens, fresh meat and fish throughout the year.

It was interesting to review the effect of gender on food preferences. No 'masculine' and 'feminine' foods, as in earlier times, were recorded. However, the larger portion of the meat was still reserved for the man, even when his main meal was late, after his return home in the evening. Yet, there were a few gender-related likes and dislikes for certain foods, with women tending to like sweets and greens, but maybe not the game or river fish, so highly appreciated by men. There was also a clear distinction in taste for drinks. If a woman drank hard liquor and especially if she did so in excess and in public, it was considered as one of the ugliest and most dishonourable acts for her family. The women preferred, or 'should prefer' less alcoholic drinks, like beer, and sweeter drinks.

Within the family, differences in taste can spark off problems or require adjustment. Men who, thanks to women, had become used to having their choices catered for, sometimes caused strife which affected the whole family, even though it was primarily aimed at those presumed responsible, i.e., the wife and/or mother. It is relevant to mention the problems faced particularly by newly weds, which were even more likely to arise when the young man had been an only son or the youngest in the family. In such cases there were sometimes problems while his new wife adapted to different culinary practices. These cooking skills, even though not generally different from those of the rest of the village women, would have had those little touches of her own mother's skills, rather than those of her mother-in-law.

As for children and adolescents, the norm is that they continue eating the traditional stews. Even so they showed some preferences that did not match what their mothers offered them. The same tastes were found again and again, and it was rare for children to like greens, offal or game. Similarly, all preferred fried eggs, steaks, hamburgers, and sausages, with chips. It was also clear that they did not dislike the stews. It was observed that in public, in the bars, etc., there was a concordance of tastes, such that some youths would choose foods they would refuse at home. In fact, each age group tried to distance itself from the group immediately junior. This wish to differentiate themselves meant that as they grew older they left behind the Coca Cola and hamburgers that they had chosen at fifteen and began to drink beer and eat *tapas* (Spanish bar snacks) until eventually they graduated to wine.

Discussion

These data, then, act to confirm the general correlation between taste and identity. Taking territorial identity first, showing a preference for local foods is an expression of unity with one's own people. In the case of cooking styles, and even in regard to basic ingredients, it is a way of showing that one takes part in local and popular ways of doing things.

The search for local identity is also felt in the villages, where they claim that the best recipes and the best flavours are found in their own typical dishes. Everyone likes to claim the invention of what is good and widely accepted, especially the great dishes placed high on the altar of gastronomic pleasures. A good example of this is ham, of which the origin and mastery are claimed by various European regions, including several Andalucian *comarcas* which produce ham. Their own is always 'the best'. What is new, on the other hand, is distrusted or rejected, except when it represents high social status, as in the case of products promoted among the young by advertising. To be aware of food and cuisine as symbols of identity is, however, relatively recent in Andalucia. Local recipe books, competitions and prizes for typical dishes, radio and television programmes, all proclaiming 'our cooking', are now multiplying and are aimed at particular audiences and supporters. Identification of a dish with one's own group and locality clearly increases the taste for it.

There is, on the other hand, another spatial aspect which is linked closely to socioeconomic status and in particular to some sectors of the working classes. I refer to migration and its relationship with food. Human mobility has caused considerable diffusion of food habits and, in association with them, of food preferences. This relates not only to the long distance transoceanic migrations, but also to internal mobility within nations. Andalucia has for centuries been an important focus of immigrants, but since the middle of the twentieth century it has been a donor population of hundreds of thousands of emigrants. These migrants have been a persistent mechanism for diffusion of food habits. The study of this, and with it of food preferences, should take into account the migratory routes and distances involved. Over the last twenty years there have been great changes in short and medium distance travel. Many of the villages in the Andalucian hills which used to receive labourers now lose them, while the coastal areas, where the new agriculture of products for export has developed, have become important centres into which farmworkers have converged. Finally, there are the longer journeys when, year after year, people from the other end of Andalucia, from Portugal and from other Iberian regions are attracted to the rural areas and the mining regions of western Andalucia. Such migrants sometimes return annually; so they mix, if not with the locals, at least with the other migratory Andalucians. This would explain, not only the similar foodstuffs, but also the similarities in the evolution of the food habits and preferences of agricultural workers from Castille, Extremadura and Andalucia.

Having to some extent discussed the geographical coordinates of taste, it is worth noting that these tend to emphasise the significance of socioeconomic position. 'Tastes ... are the practical affirmation of an inevitable difference' wrote Bourdieu (1979), the affirmation and establishment of which are produced through distancing oneself from or discarding other tastes. Thus, the certainty, and even vehemence, with which taste can be expressed becomes one of the most important barriers that arise between different social classes. Tastes unite those who share them and distance those who do not. They cause a fundamental barrier that separates the 'tastes of luxury' and the 'tastes of necessity' (Bourdieu, 1979: 55-6).

However, the manner in which the configuration of taste is articulated will depend in the first instance on the particular social structure of each case. In rural Andalucia, the scarcity in the villages of the artistocracy and of the mercantile upper classes provides little opportunity for the manifestations of refined taste and, therefore, little opportunity for social differentiation. The nobles, who represented the most superior levels of taste and who even today are up to a point the 'dance masters of Europe', as Karl Marx wrote, do not live in the villages. The upper echelons of the merchant classes, who have been the principal players responsible for the important changes that have occurred in European kitchens, especially in big cities, hardly exist here and where they do they have tastes closer to those that are local and popular than to cosmopolitan refinements. The middle classes, for their part, provide the first step for the wider distribution of tastes since, as Bourdieu put it, the poorest classes understand taste as a form of negation, or opposition to others. 'As for the working classes, perhaps their sole function in the system of aesthetic positions is to serve as a foil, a negative reference point, in relation to which all aesthetics define themselves, by successive negations' (Bourdieu, 1979: 57). In this way, a more or less lineal cline is produced in peoples' aspirations.

In nutrition, it is possible to make a distinction between essential needs, those that satisfy biological necessities, and the relative needs, those which might be seen to depend either on a set of failures of satisfaction or on a search for a taste which is more pleasant or, in some significant way, more élitist. In this sense, one can differentiate between basic senses of well-being, remembering that all exist in their own space and time and, as such, are variable. As far as those associated with luxury, reserved for the minority, are concerned, they cannot be controlled. Finally there are those useless fruits of the consumer society, that, even though they now reach all, are sold as if only a few priviledged individuals could attain them. In the case of the Andalucia of today, ham and shellfish represent just such widespread 'luxuries' of the consumer society. They are products for a huge 'minority'. These foods have been produced for all, but are purchased principally by the middle classes, who, more than the rest of the community, appear never to be satisfied. This provokes their constant need to consume and consume. They wish for more and better foods. Meanwhile, the lower classes' preference for the essentials can be defined negatively as an opposition to these other foods. Such concepts end up making their own reality. A voluntary choice – an act of liberty – is created out of a state of necessity. It is tempting to include a few more lines by Bourdieu: 'the art of drinking and eating remains one of the few areas in which the working classes explicitly challenge the legitimate art of living' (Bourdieu, 1979: 179).

This theme has been demonstrated throughout this research; all members of domestic groups in the lower classes confirmed that what they most liked to eat was precisely what they did eat. This general conformity does not mean that they are not conscious of what they can attain and what they cannot. Sailors know very well which fish are 'good' and which are not so good, but they also know that they can seldom have the best fish on their own tables. In the same way, the traditional stew, with all its correct ingredients[1] is not as common as labourers would like in their homes. However, they are generally satisfied and would not change their daily food. It does not occur to them to say that they would like more ham or more shellfish, even though they probably would. They buy these things for celebrations and seem to understand that these delicacies are reserved only for certain occasions. So, in contrast to the middle classes, day-to-day meals are not the time for more expensive foods, but the time to enjoy the well-known and familiar flavours of all of one's life.

In fact, out of that rejection of those foods which they cannot attain on a regular basis, (frequently those which others desire but also do not always achieve) they make necessity a voluntary choice. One should not forget that these sectors of the Andalucian population are descended from generations of people burdened with food scarcity and even hunger. For example, the experiences of the 1940s, after the Spanish Civil War, still linger in the memories of many. So, the food habits of the unsalaried majority of the population evolved in a similar manner to become those of most rural Andalucian regions. These habits have now consolidated into very stable 'tastes', repeated over generations and learnt from infancy. The identification of the majority of the population with these popular and traditional tastes has been converted into an important element in the collective definition of the identity itself. It is held in contrast to more refined tastes and definitely in defiance of the symbols of social distinction to which they have no access. In summary, and as in the

---

1. In Andalucia when talking of the *avios del cocido* (for the stew) they mean that meat, bones and dried salt pork or beef are included.

case of local differences, each social class sees its own food preferences and tastes as natural and correct.

To return to the effects of age, because of its interaction with eco-
nomics for poorer people, the differences of taste between age
cohorts seem, at first glance, highly important. More detailed analysis, however, of the data obtained in this study offers a less clear
vision of the evolution of food habits across cohorts. Also observed
was a tendency to turn to foods which had been rejected by a
younger age group. For example, when youths join the labour market and begin their own families, they see themselves obliged to
adopt less controversial food habits. One must not forget that the
stews and other traditional foods provide an economic form of adequate nutrition. Since in the street people go on trying foods that
they do not eat at home, the bars become ritualised places for tasting
new things. There they try chops, snails and other dishes they would
scorn at home.

Another topic, frequently referred to, is the importance of advertising in the development of preferences, above all among young
people. In the case of Andalucia, the seduction of advertising is interwoven with the historical event of overcoming food scarcity – a
scarcity which those who lived through it find hard to forget. Change
has been very rapid and the possibility of choosing between many
foods is recent. In only three decades, there has been a marked
increase in the variety along the shelves of supermarkets, in contrast
to the centuries when only scarcity and misery were known. An
apparent gap has opened up between the harsh realities remem-
bered by old people and the experiences of those under thirty. The
former have witnessed the change and the latter live as though people have always revelled in *la abundancia*. Furthermore, young people tend to try to imitate the current fashions found in other, more
industrialised, countries, but their economic possibilities are far from
unlimited. The indices of unemployment are very high in Andalucia
and for many products an optimum quality/price relationship has
not yet been found. An example of this is found in the fact that the
mass-produced cakes and biscuits, with trade names popular with
children, are not eaten so frequently in those villages where local
cooperatives still produce, at a low price, the traditional pastries.

These days young people from a relatively early age reject the
food of older people. It is a form of independence from parental
authority and culture (James, 1979). However, there is no reason to
believe that these modern youths have discovered a new world.
When there is little to eat, the food of the old people tastes much better than when there are plenty of other things to choose from. It is

very likely that the majority of the younger generation will one day rediscover their taste for most of the foods that they now reject, even if not all. It seems, however, unlikely that those dishes on which the mother traditionally spent many hours in preparation will be retained or restored.

Conclusion

Taste in foods has, then, the capacity to become an instrument of identity, be it of age, gender, socioeconomic status, ethnicity or religion. Thus it demonstrates differences and creates barriers between groups. However, above all else, taste is, as Toussaint-Samat wrote (1991: 150) 'a combination of physical sensations, but at the same time a conceptual activity, an analysis, in summary an intellectual act'. It should not be forgotten that taste for a given food or dish is forged through the conflation of flavour, texture, consistency, smell, etc. Very many physical sensations are received, interpreted and analysed within, and in relation to, the position that each person has in the world, and their perception of this position.

There is no doubt but that cultural aspects are very important when the palate is being formed. Taste may indeed be a primary pleasure, learned from infancy and bonded to the maternal world in the first place. However, while developing, it becomes a fundamental process of interpretation of reality, through which new models are approached and reflected in certain types of foods, or, as usually occurs, a re-identification with one's own world: the mother, the place, the social group, the village and the region.

In all cases, very deep-rooted and internalised preferences, developed through slow, poorly understood evolution, are involved. In this way it can be perceived why different ethnocentric reactions to food are so frequent and immediate. Taste also occupies a difficult position of balance between reality and desire. Affected by its own evolution it is found just at that intermediate point between that food which one covets and that which one actually gets to eat.

However, in spite of the importance of cultural aspects, there exists an upper limit in what is viable in the study of taste from an anthropological point of view. It is still not known precisely how all tastes work physiologically. What are the real possibilities for assimilation of the many new flavours that the food industries are likely to offer in the future? Will there exist a tendency to assimilate them into familiar patterns? Will it be the intensity that dominates? Not only is there still much to discover about the exact way in which the human body works, but also it is essential to study the relevant cultures and differences within cultures. So, once more it is important to recommend collaboration between different disciplines for a theme as complex as food preferences.

References

Bourdieu, P. (1979) *Distinction: A Social Critique of the Judgement of Taste* (Trans. R. Nice), Routledge & Kegan Paul, London

Florencio, A. and Lopez, A.L. (1933) Migraciones estacionales y mercado de trabajo en la Baja Andalucia de la primera mitad del siglo, XIX, *Proceedings of the Congresso de la Asociación de Demografía Histórica*, Santiago de Compostela

González Turmo, I. (1992) La Pêche fluvial dans le bas Guadalquivir (Espagne), *Anthropologies Maritimes*, 4: 119-28

James, A. (1979) Confections, concoctions and conceptions, *Journal of the Anthropological Society of Oxford*, 10(2): 83-95

Toussaint-Samat, M. (1991) *Historia Natural y Moral de los Alimentos*, Alianza, Madrid, 5: 72

10. EVOLUTION IN EATING HABITS IN THE ALTO DOURO OF NORTHERN PORTUGAL

Manuela Valagao

Introduction

If the social changes which have occurred in Portugal during the past three decades have modified the traditional eating habits (Valagao, 1989a), the rural areas are no doubt the places where the impact of different phenomena of change should be most evident. Although inequalities are not visible in data on consumption levels, analysis of the evolution of food availability in Portugal during the period 1960 to 1980 shows a pattern of considerable increase in milk, meat, vegetable oils, sugar, soft drinks and beer consumption. For example, milk consumption increased 181 percent, meat 151 percent (chicken having reached 1,279 percent!), soft drinks 747 percent and beer 788 percent (Valagao, 1989a). For the period 1980 to 1990, there are no available data using a similar methodology. In rural areas the content, number, timing, duration and context of meals have undergone substantial changes. These changes appear to be a consequence of new patterns of time management and different lifestyles, which have both become increasingly like urban patterns. This chapter is primarily concerned with the very recent development of food diversity in the poor labouring class in a rural part of Portugal. Food diversity is an important precursor for food preferences, because only in the relative luxury of food choices can preferences be expressed.

I shall attempt to define the connection between these changes and food preferences in a well identified area and time span. The region is the Alto Douro of the northern interior of Portugal, and it covers roughly the demarcated area for production of Port wine, classified by the European Community as a 'top quality wine'. Of all the rural populations of Portugal, the traditional living conditions of those in the Alto Douro were known to be the worst, and that even in the richest agricultural area of Portugal! (Lima Basto and de Barros, 1943).

To understand this evolution better, I refer to a key period in Portugal's recent social and economic history, i.e., the years between the 1960s and 1980s. During this period, the most important changes in the study area are, on the one hand, the interrelation between working patterns and the changes in content, time and duration of meals, and, on the other hand, the diversification of eating habits within the family. Only with these changes has there been any possibility of diversity in food preferences, for as González Turmo (this volume) discusses, the preferences of the poorest are expressed in terms of sufficiency of what is available to them and what they are used to.

Poverty and Wealth

In the Alto Douro the landscape and agriculture are ruled by the seasonal cycle of the grapevine. In this famous Port wine area, all local life has been organised around its production, a most important feature of the Portuguese economy (Barreto, 1988; Martins, 1988). The spread of vineyards dates back to the late eighteenth century and is a result of a monocultural system. Since that period, the vine has become the central focus of the landscape, economy, and society (Barreto, 1988) whose identity can only be perceived by means of this all-pervading feature. The wine producing activity takes place in an institutional framework, which sets very strict rules, and it has been this way since 1756, when the Alto Douro was established as a *Regiao Demarcada* for the production of quality wine. We have here the oldest *Appelation d'Origine Controllé* in the world.

Monoculture frequently leads to a polarisation of the social hierarchy. At the one extreme, there is a very high social status for the few, and, at the other, a very low social status for the many. The working classes used to be totally dependent on those for whom they worked, and today the local population recalls life in the 1940s and 1950s in terms of slavery, poverty, squalor, and describes a complete dependence on the 'bosses' represented locally by their foremen (Pereira, 1941). These men had the power to decide who was going to work and who was not. The same applied to the small-scale wine producers who were victims of any slump in demand for Port wine (Martins, 1988) and who also lived below the poverty level. A small producer now in his late fifties, referred to 'houses that were not real houses but shacks made of dried mud'. He continued, 'as for any work, it was up to the boss. In those days the workers, hat in hand, would wait for the boss to come out of Sunday mass. On Monday morning, their hoe on their shoulder, they would beg for work. Whether they would get it or not was "God's will" and they had to accept it'.

In such a system, a strong structure of domination arose; the wealth of the 'masters', owners of large estates and/or of large Port wineries, existed beside the extreme poverty of the other inhabitants of Alto Douro, be they small wine growers or farm labourers. Living exclusively on vine growing, the inhabitants of this traditionally agricultural area saw their income become dependent on the price of the wine and its marketing system, widening further the gap between the two poles of society. Estate owners only came to Alto Douro at harvest time, and the locals recall their wealth and luxurious lifestyle through, among other things, the lavish banquets served in the *quintas* (estates) to the various guests during their yearly visit (Torga, 1947). At such events, the table was a place of celebration, of the pleasures of eating and drinking. The menus showed a rich variety of dishes and desserts (Vizetelly, 1947; Torga, 1947), some even borrowed from other regions or countries, demonstrating the close similarity of tastes among equivalent élite groups around Europe.

At the other end of the scale, for small producers and labourers, soup was the staple food. This was a one course meal, served on all occasions. It consisted of vegetables and a small quantity of salted meat boiled at length, with no great variation from day to day. The agricultural produce was consumed locally (Pereira, 1941) and there was very little circulation of currency. Until the 1960s it was only through a great deal of hard work and the endurance of real hardship that the majority of inhabitants were able to survive, keeping to this dull frugal diet, similar to that of peasants in mediæval Provence, based on cabbage, beans and fat bacon (Stouff, 1970; Claudian and Serville, 1970), which also remained unchanged for centuries because of the immobility of the majority in a poor terrain.

Thus, the close link between social hierarchy and eating habits (Grignon, 1980; 1986) shows a sharp contrast between wealth and poverty, marking until very recently the distinctive character of the area.

The Crucial Years: 1960 to 1980

During these twenty years, the area witnessed small but widespread changes. First, the work force started to decrease because of the economic boom and the reconstruction of northern Europe, which provoked an intensified migration (Valagao, 1989b) towards that area. Then war broke out in the Portuguese colonies of Africa and men left for the army. Within the country, the growing importance of factory work and services allowed the younger generations access to a less strenuous way of life. The poor standard of living in rural areas, so far taken for granted, was being questioned. In 1962, a revolt by peasants in the Alentejo (east central Portugal) led to the introduction of a Bill enforcing the eight-hour working day. The Alto Douro, without means of communication with Alentejo, did not benefit from this, but it was nevertheless the sign of a process which had started to gain ground. From the early 1960s onwards, the first Port wine cooperatives were established in Alto Douro, freeing the small-scale producers from dependence on wine merchants. This trend remained marginal at first, until the grape growers in large numbers joined together in cooperatives in the late 1960s, revealing an urge for autonomy (Lema, 1980).

When former inhabitants of the Alto Douro who had emigrated or gone to the wars, returned to their native area, they brought with them new requirements in food preferences and eating habits. This is well illustrated in local life histories, as in the case of a forty-eight year-old ex-emigrant to France, currently a small-scale vine grower. He explained why he left the country after his return from the Angola war in 1967: 'you know, you can't accept this poverty when you have seen other worlds; I came back from over there where I could even afford to drink beer, and here it remained the same old story, every day broth and corn bread; I couldn't put up with it and there was something in the back of my mind that made me want things to be different'. Transformations were slowly taking shape, but not until the Portuguese Revolution of 1974 was the will to change clearly expressed. After that date, the changes became apparent, drawing the Alto Douro slowly but steadily into the 1980s.

The changes taking place in the area during the 1970s were part of a vast economic boom in Portugal, found also in the rest of Europe. The distribution network of Port and other wines increased to meet new demands, both national and international (Barreto, 1988; Martins, 1988). Industry and services in full expansion began to employ workers on a large scale, offering better salaries and less strenuous work. This was bound to modify the living conditions of the rural population in the Alto Douro. The number of those working exclusively on the land had reduced, but agricultural activity did not decrease, and the rural characteristics of the area were reinforced in regard to the monoculture of the vine. It did, however, lead to the abandonment of grain production (corn and rye), which was not economically viable, and resulted in the disappearance of home-made bread (Valagao, 1990). This explains the change in the type of bread consumed: the need to buy it led to the widespread consumption of wheat bread which in the past had been rare and confined to festive occasions. The revolution of 1974 created the circumstances for extremely important social reforms, particularly for the rural population of the Alto Douro; for example, the introduction of compulsory education and various welfare benefits such as maternity leave and crêche facilities. There was a new window on the outside world with the advent of television, as the locals put it: 'it has brought Lisbon's luxury goods and other fine things to us'. Through advertising, the peasants became familiar with consumer goods previously unknown to them. The eight-hour working day was adopted, an increasing number of producers joined the cooperatives and the women had access to salaried employment. Life in the Alto Douro had changed, as witnessed also by the widespread use of currency among the locals.

However, to witness a radical change in eating habits and food preferences in general, we have to wait until the 1980s, when the effect of all those social changes became perceptible (Valagao, 1987). In that decade, the availability of new consumer goods, the modernisation of kitchen equipment and utensils and the introduction of the freezer as a method of preservation, promoted a true revolution in food patterns and behaviour.

Changes Related to Food and Work

As explained above, working and eating patterns had remained substantially unchanged until well into the 1960s. Labour was in rhythm with the seasons, which meant toiling from dawn to dusk. The image of poverty of peasant life in the area is reinforced by climatic data: very cold winters and hot summers. Locally they say 'nine months of winter and three of Hell'. There is a lack of accurate information on meal times and duration, and I can only make an estimate. It would necessarily depend on the urgency of the work, which was in turn dependent on the season.

In winter, work started at dawn, but as the sun rose later, the breakfast break would take place at around nine o'clock. Dinner time was around 12.15 pm. The time of the evening meal or supper depended of course on the various work patterns set by the seasons and the availability of food. It depended also on whether or not it was the season for the afternoon snack, known locally as the *merenda*, because the time of day and period of the year set for the *merenda* was strictly coded. The period between 25 March, 'Our Lady of the Merendas' day, and 5 September, 'Our Lady of Remedios' day, was the most strenuous work period of the year, and those meal breaks were fully justified. Except for the evening meal and for Sundays, all other meals were taken at the place of work, out in the vineyards, if the weather would allow it. If it rained or snowed, the workers remained at home without work and without pay. The meal composition would fit these circumstances. This pattern had remained unchanged for centuries, (Novonha, 1942; Torga, 1947) with the *almoço* (breakfast or 'morning lunch'), *jantar* (dinner) and *ceia* (supper), consisting of very much the same foods and following their seasonal availability.

The social and economic changes described above had a considerable impact on this traditional pattern, because of a complete alteration of living and working conditions. For those working in factories or service industries, the midday meal was changed from the old peasant soup or bean dishes and acquired a new emphasis, richer in meat and fish. In those families where even the women now worked exclusively in the fields, there was much less time than in the past for housework and cooking. Women, therefore, opted for foods that took a shorter amount of time to prepare and cook. Apart from farm labourers who still have their meals in the vineyards or fields, all others now have their midday meals at home, at the local restaurant or at the work canteen. For these, leisure time has become a new reality. It is usually spent in the local bar, over a glass of beer. In Santa Marta de Penaguiao, a district of the Alto Douro, between 1980 and 1987 the number of bars has increased from seventeen to sixty-two and the number of cafés has risen from five to thirty (Valagao, 1990).

With individual changes in time management and the rising purchasing power of the households, the eating habits that were so homogeneous in the past have been altered, changing the traditional preparation and consumption of food in the family circle. This change from homogeneity based perhaps on timetables means variety and choice, which in turn provides the opportunity for the expression of preferences.

Changes in Food Habits

The link between meal structure and the way people manage their time becomes clear in the coexistence of different eating habits within the same family. And we see here that the changing food patterns and preferences within a population during a given period in a given place, relate to a whole variety of recent transformations in lifestyles and goes far beyond the simple expression of individual needs and tastes. The simultaneous existence of all the differences reflects the shift from old and well-established rules to new ones still in the making. If 'the vine sets the rules' as they say in Douro, then the work patterns deriving from it no longer represent the central focus around which food patterns are organised. It is a clear demonstration of cultural evolution.

The most important change so far has been that the people in the Alto Douro today eat when they are hungry; all families can now afford to do so. Furthermore the content of the meals has changed both through the diversity of foods available and the introduction of products with which the locals were previously not acquainted (dairy products, meat products, coffee and cocoa by-products), and because of the new availability of foods which they had always known about but which they had previously had little access to because of cost (meat, wheat bread, fish and fresh fruit).

Until the 1960s the consumption of dairy products was practically nonexistent. It then started to become a regular feature and is now part of the morning meal of almost every child. The diversification of food products enables children to eat alone, at home, nibbling all day, when in the past serving the morning soup and the stews had been a family occasion. Previously, everyone shared the same foods and the same life. Today, the coexistence of different generations within the family imposes a new diversity of eating schedules. During the week, everyone manages his/her meals according to his/her needs and tastes.

Besides the alterations in meal content, there are fundamental changes to commensality. The morning meal is now eaten according to individual wishes and obligations. It ranges from a hefty meal taken at 9.00 am by farm labourers, including soup (and the use of a fork), to an early breakfast of no more than coffee and milk, taken earlier by those who go off to school or to the factory. The name given to the midday meal depends on the particular circumstances of individuals: dinner for those working in the fields, but lunch for those who go to school or follow an urban pattern. As we see, the time and type of meal can differ widely between individual members of the same family. The greatest fluctuations are seen in the time of the midday meal, especially among the children and young people who have to fit into the 'school shift system', i.e., the current school practice of concentrating classes into the morning or the afternoon, and among the women who increasingly participate in wine production. A large number of wives of small producers have taken over from their husbands, and since this affects, among other things, meal timing and preparation, the time spent cooking has been considerably reduced over the past ten years. There is therefore a dwindling importance of the old soup staple, which is now confined to a very secondary place.

The evening meal has also changed, due to the secondary activities available to everyone after a normal working day. Traditionally, the whole family would gather together for supper. Now, since there are opportunities for taking a walk, visiting the local bar, or working in one's own vegetable garden or vineyard, the various members of the family will eat that meal at different times. There is also a seasonal factor linked to this: in winter, there are more opportunities for everyone to meet for supper, since work in the vineyards is less time consuming.

However, the most important change in the recent past concerns the *merenda* or mid-afternoon snack which was linked to the old working conditions. The local point of view is that it has ceased to exist in its traditional sense, as the dawn-to-dusk work in the fields no longer happens, but this kind of afternoon snack has been changed into another type of meal which takes place at home (no longer in the vineyard) and has come to signify a pause between two types of activity in the afternoon. It has become the transition between work taking place in the factory or the office and the more domestic 'work' in one's own vineyard or vegetable garden.

Change, yet Continuity

The transformation of certain elements is not incompatible with the permanence of others. The diversity of eating habits analysed above is unified by a series of more constant features, and it is suggested that the changes have not altered a certain continuity. The techniques for food preparation remain the same, the dishes for which the family will gather around the table are still stews, leaving the roast, which had been very rare in the past, to star now as the Sunday dish. Food sharing, when it takes place around the family table, follows traditional rules: the choicest pieces must be given to the men, husbands and sons, who are still considered to work the hardest outside the home. They deserve different treatment since they are the ones 'who earn the money'.

Changes in the children's eating patterns have been particularly great: dairy products, wheat bread, cornflakes and other new types of food are now viewed as essential products for them. However, they tend to have an unbalanced diet, too rich in sugars and carbohydrates, because they now are able to indulge in their taste for these things. They are constantly nibbling when at home, without the control of a maternal presence, as the mother is busy both with a variety of jobs outside the home and attending to all the different needs of her family at home.

As explained above, the *merenda* has not disappeared, it is a replacement in an existing continuum. It has a different context, identified now with the idea of freedom and pleasure. It asserts pride in land ownership 'where one works when one wants to' and these factors are reflected in the more diversified composition of this meal. It consists mainly of highly prized products, such as fish preserves, ham and other meat products. It has become a symbol of the availability of what were once scarce and expensive foods, and of a freedom to choose, which had been totally unknown for these people only twenty years ago.

Conclusion

The chronological framework of the social changes identified in this paper is closely linked to the evolution of daily life in the Alto Douro, and these include eating habits and the development of food preferences.

Small and medium sized wine producers now tend to take main jobs in factories or services, and their work in the vineyards has become one of free choice rather than compulsory toil. This acquired freedom brings about a greater diversity in eating habits. A further fact is that notwithstanding a dwindling paid work force, the monoculture of the vine has expanded. This has been made possible because women have been able to take on their share of vine work because of the introduction of a new diet and the adoption of cooking methods which require less time than in the past.

Even if change has occurred with regard to food patterns and consumption it does not imply a suppression of the past, and an interesting and paradoxical situation is therefore created: the fast adoption of food habits, which are closer to an urban model, coexists with the traditional and well-known practices of the rural situation. Modernity and tradition are both a reality in the Alto Douro of today.

This framework is an essential feature, since over barely twenty years the Alto Douro has undergone a series of profound changes. It is a very short time for such an evolution. This evolution is the setting within which, with new choices now available, a rural population is learning the more affluent concept of food preferences.

Acknowledgement

My thanks go to Annie Hubert for her editorial suggestions.

References

Barreto, A. (1988) O vinho do Porto e a intervencao do estado, *Analise Social*, XXIV (100): 373-90

Claudian, J. and Serville, Y (1970) Les aliments du dimanche et du vendredi: Etudes sur le comportement alimentaire actuel en France, in J.J.Hemardinquer, *Aspects de l'evolution recente du comportement alimentaire en France: composition des repas et 'urbanisation'*, Armand Colin, Paris, 300-6

Grignon, C. and Ch. (1980) Styles d'alimentation et gouts popularies, *Revue Francaise de Sociologie*, XX: 4

Grignon, C. and Ch. (1986) Practiques alimentaires et classes sociales, *Rev. problemes politiques et sociaux*, No. 544, Paris

Lema, P.B. (1980) *O Alto Douro,* Estudios de Geografia Humana e Regional, Centro de Estudos Geograficos da Universidade de Lisboa, INIC, Lisbon

Lima Basto, E.A. (1935) *Niveis de vida e custo de vida, o caso do operario agricola portgues,* Separata do volume, Conferencias realizadas no ano lectivo de 1935-1936, Univ.Tecnica de Lisboa, ISA, Lisbon

Lima Basto, E.A. and de Barros H. (1943) *Inquerito a habitacao rural* (promovido pelo Senado Universitario), Vol. I, in Minho, Douro Litoral, Tras-os-Montes e Alto-Douro *A Habiacao Rural nas Provincias do Norte de Portgual*), Lisboa

Martins, C.A. (1988) Os ciclos do vinho do Porto: ensaio de periodizacao, *Analise Social,* XXIV(100), 391-429

Noronha, R. de (1942) *Alimentaca dos rurais do Douro- Subsidios para um estudo medico-social* (Conferencia proferida em 29 de Maio de 1942 no Clube dos Fenianos Portuenses, a convite da Liga Portuguesa de Profilaxia Social), Regua, Imprensa do Douro

Pereira, M.B. (1941) Preparacao para o estudo de um valor economico, *Anais do Instituto do Vinho do Porto,* No.2, Porto, 443-54

Stouff, L. (1970) *Ravitaillement et alimentation en Provence au XIVe et XVe siecles,* Paris, Ecole Practique des Hautes Etudes, Paris

Torga, M. (1947) *Vindima,* Ed. do Autor, Coimbra

Valagao, M.M. and Baptista, M.P. (1981) Consumo e habitos alimentares de um grupo de familias rurais no concelho de Ponte de Lima, *Revista CEN,* 5(3), Nov. Lisbon

Valagao, M.M. (1987) *Consumo e habitos alimentares de um grupo de familias rurais no Alto-Douro,* DEESA/INIA, No. 9, Lisboa

Valagao, M.M. (1989a) A situacao alimentar em Portgual, *Revista Portuguesa de Nutricao,* 1(1): 15-26

Valagao, M.M. (1989b) Practicas alimentares dos emigrantes: Mudanca ou continuidade?, *Revista sociedade e territorio,* 8, Afrontamento, Porto

Valagao, M.M. (1990) *Praticas alimentares numa sociedade em Mudanca: estudo de caso numa frequesia do Alto Douro,* Tese de doutoramento, FCT/ Universidade Nova de Lisboa

Vizetelly, H. (1947) *No pais do vinho do Porto* (traducao de *Facts about Porto and Madeira,* 1887), Porto, Inst. Vinho do Porto, Porto

11. NATIONALITY AND FOOD PREFERENCES IN THE CERDANYA VALLEY, EASTERN PYRENES

Helen Macbeth and *Alex Green*

Introduction

This chapter concerns a study of food preferences in two samples of teenagers either side of the Franco-Spanish border. It reveals results of potential interest not only to anthropologists and food purveyors, but also to human biologists and epidemiologists because food choices affect nutrition and the body's biology.

That the aetiology of food preferences is multifactorial is made clear by the topics covered in this book. Over the last fifteen years, there has been increased interest in children's development of such preferences (e.g., Petersen et al., 1984; Sundberg and Endres, 1984; Rosen and Silberg, 1988; Jeanneret, 1989; Rozin, 1990). Several studies (e.g., Birch, 1988; Alles-White and Welch, 1985) have given strong support to the idea that food preferences are formed while children are very young. Others view the development as continuing over a longer period. Court's (1988) paper provides a useful summary of research on the topic as it applies to teenagers, but James (1979) provided an interesting perspective on the separate culture of teenagers and how this can be signalled in their food choices. It is clear that the food and drink manufacturers and their advertisers are well aware of this subculture of teenagers, who attempt to conform to a concept of their own peer group in contrast to that of the adults around them. It

is also well known that television advertising influences children's
choices (e.g., Galst and White, 1976; Goldberg, Gorn and Gibson,
1978; Dietz, 1990). Although frequently deplored (see e.g., Story,
1990), much advertising is about food and drink (Peck, 1979) and is
obviously directed at children and teenagers. Television is not the
only source of such advertising, which is also colourfully represented
on billboards and in magazines. The similarity of such advertise-
ments around Europe (and in the United States and Australia)
demonstrates the power of the multinational companies and one
might expect that a teenager subculture is now international (Walker,
1996). This is certainly a believable situation when one observes
teenager clothing. If so, teenagers in different countries would have
more food preferences in common than do their elders.

As part of a biosocial study in a Pyrenean valley, dissected by the
Franco-Spanish border, the food preferences of teenagers were
explored with a view to comparing those from the French side and
those from the Spanish side. The study was part of a larger research
project on the similarity or otherwise of lifestyles with a view to
analysing non-genetic effects on human biology. A study of food
intake frequencies demonstrated significant differences (Macbeth,
1992; Macbeth, 1995). It was expected that even a small study of
teenager attitudes would throw light on the development of lifestyle
differences. Our research in this valley began with a study of the
marriage registers in every parish, French and Spanish. From these
records it was established that over the years 1915 to 1984 there had
been sufficient frequency of transfrontier marriages to make detection of any heterogeneity in gene frequencies most unlikely (Macbeth, Salvat, Vigo and Bertranpetit, 1996). With this presumption of
genetic homogeneity, any differences in teenage food preferences
became twice as interesting because of the clearer demonstration
that differences must be learned.

The valley to be discussed is by no means isolated as more than
one trans-Pyrenean route traverse it and it is the destination of holi-
daymakers, many with holiday homes. The valley lies in the eastern
Pyrenees within the region that was, in the thirteenth century, united
in one kingdom, Catalonia, but is now divided between the nation
states of France and Spain (Sahlins, 1989). Called Cerdanya in Catalan, Cerdagne in French and Cerdaña in Castilian Spanish, the valley experiences diverse cultures and yet has a unity in its geography
and in its multiculturalism. Individual residents may refer to themselves as Catalan, French or Spanish, and many will claim to be Catalan *and* French or Spanish, and even announce their *Cerdan* loyalties
as well. It is a relatively wide and sunny valley with green pastures

that has attracted competition, frequently military, over the centuries. Our interest lies in the division between two nation states of a valley, physically united by surrounding mountains. The further perspective of the common Catalan ethnicity, identified by many locals, adds yet another dimension at a time when *nationality* and *ethnicity* are important topics within Europe (Macbeth and Bertranpetit, 1995).

Method

The one formal border crossing, with customs officers and police regularly on duty, lies between two adjacent towns, Puigcerdá on the Spanish side and Bourg Madame on the French, whose outskirts now touch at this border post and whose centres lie barely four kilometres apart. On the French side, for the age group eleven to fifteen years, there is in Bourg Madame one state school, *le Collège*, but on the Spanish side there is an age division of schools at thirteen years. Those under thirteen in Puigcerdá go to Alfons Primer, the primary school. Then for those over thirteen, there is a further division between the "Institut" and the Escola Professional, the latter providing more practical courses. All the schools involved had much wider catchment areas than the limits of the two towns. So, school children from quite isolated rural areas were brought together with those who lived in the towns. Some from rural areas lived closer to neighbours across the border than to the school they went to.

Permission was granted by the directors of each school for the main researcher to interview the children within a class situation. In total 664 children took part; 345 Spanish children and 319 French children successfully completed a questionnaire on preferences and concepts about health values of certain food items. Table 11.1 shows the total number of pupils from each school who took part in our preference survey. Very few were absent; two decided not to participate. In this paper, nationality is determined simply by the school attended by each child. This was considered more appropriate than trying to identify cases of recent and not so recent migration across the border.

After a brief introduction about food and nutrition to each class in each school, a questionnaire was handed to each pupil. The questionnaire contains a list of foods followed by several columns. The first four columns correspond to the levels of preferences: *I like it very much; I like it; indifferent; I don't like it;* and children were asked to put a cross in the relevant column, beside each foodstuff in turn. The next three columns correspond to the child's view of whether frequent consumption of that food was: *healthy; indifferent; unhealthy.*

Table 11.1 Number of pupils participating from each school

		ALL	M	F
France	Le Collège	319	170	149
Spain	Alfons Primer	218	105	113
	el Institut	76	32	44
	la Escola Professional	51	28	23

The choice of foods was governed to some extent by a previous little study in La Rioja (Castro, 1991), but was modified to highlight foods of interest in the study of coronary heart disease. In the event no comparison with the Rioja study was valid as the latter turned out to be excessively small, and more independent thought could have been given to a choice of food items to concur better with other parts of the Cerdanya research. Because of the authors' amazement at seeing school children smoke quite openly in the Spanish schools, the non-food item 'cigarettes' was included to see what the response would be.

A relatively restricted time was allowed and respondents were asked not to discuss answers with neighbours, a request which was for the most part enforced by teachers and so observed. However, as it was a break from normal school work, a generally cheerful atmosphere reigned. There were occasional outbreaks of hilarity, some caused by the British researcher's use of their language, and this may have affected a few answer sheets. Owing to time constraints a slightly smaller sample completed the health attitudes section.

Answers in the preference and health columns were then coded numerically and in this paper analysis has been limited to calculating frequencies in each column on each side of the border and chi-square (X^2) calculations to check the significance of differences between the answers of the Spanish and the French children for each food item listed.

Results

As an introduction to results, Tables 11.2 and 11.3 show the crosstabulation and X^2 results. While on the questionnaire food items were deliberately arranged in no logical order, in the tables they are grouped for easier reference to the discussion. In Table 11.2, after the

Table 11.2 Food preferences expressed by Spanish and French teenagers

Item	Nation	Not Like	Indifferent	Like	Like V.M.	X^2	Sig.
Wholemeal bread	S	31.2	30.1	26.4	12.3		
	F	14.0	21.5	35.2	29.3	54.11	***
Sunflower oil	S	19.9	55.5	23.7	0.8		
	F	11.9	48.8	35.0	4.4	14.03	**
Olive oil	S	11.6	38.2	43.2	7.1		
	F	22.1	30.7	38.7	8.6	9.06	*
Margarine	S	25.5	37.0	27.2	10.3		
	F	30.1	37.0	24.8	8.2	n.s.	
Butter	S	17.5	32.2	36.5	13.8		
	F	10.7	26.3	45.1	17.9	12.27	**
Milk	S	5.4	7.7	29.3	57.5		
	F	7.1	7.5	25.2	60.2	n.s.	
Yoghurt	S	4.3	8.8	35.3	51.6		
	F	2.8	6.0	38.9	52.4	n.s.	
Water	S	1.5	9.1	42.4	47.1		
	F	0.6	9.3	38.6	51.4	n.s.	
Meats and Fish							
Pork	S	15.3	28.2	38.3	18.2		
	F	13.8	27.4	42.8	16.0	n.s.	
Lamb	S	9.7	18.3	42.0	30.0		
	F	21.5	18.6	35.3	24.6	18.66	***
Hamburgers	S	10.8	10.8	37.9	40.5		
	F	14.2	12.6	23.0	50.3	17.61	***
Liver	S	51.9	18.2	17.1	12.8		
	F	41.9	11.3	25.9	20.9	21.77	***
Rabbit	S	12.5	16.5	40.1	31.0		
	F	9.7	14.3	39.3	36.8	n.s.	
Tuna	S	8.4	21.6	40.1	30.0		
	F	6.6	17.3	38.4	37.7	n.s.	
Cod	S	40.2	28.0	20.5	11.3		
	F	45.9	20.4	22.6	11.1	n.s.	
Hake	S	24.0	29.5	30.3	16.2		
	F	30.7	23.0	24.2	22.0	10.49	*
Vegetables and Fruit							
Cabbage	S	49.7	25.4	16.0	8.9		
	F	34.9	23.3	32.1	9.7	27.23	***
Greens	S	27.3	25.9	28.4	18.5		
	F	16.9	19.4	33.9	29.8	21.62	***
Spinach	S	46.9	20.9	19.7	12.6		
	F	38.4	14.7	22.5	24.4	19.73	***
Lettuce	S	9.1	18.0	33.1	39.7		
	F	16.0	12.3	33.6	38.1	10.10	*
Lentils	S	21.1	24.0	32.9	22.0		
	F	13.4	16.1	38.8	31.7	18.52	***
Chickpeas	S	28.0	33.4	26.9	11.7		
	F	25.2	22.1	29.0	23.7	22.13	***

Table 11.2 *Continued*

Item	Nation	Not Like	Indifferent	Like	Like V.M.	X^2	Sig.
Rice	S	0.9	13.5	49.0	36.7		
	F	2.2	11.4	46.0	40.3		n.s.
Apples	S	3.7	11.7	42.6	42.0		
	F	0.6	6.9	43.5	48.9	12.83	**
Oranges	S	4.9	9.2	34.4	51.6		
	F	4.1	5.6	36.3	54.1		n.s.
Fruit Juice	S	0.9	5.1	21.4	72.6		
	F	0.9	2.8	20.5	75.8		n.s.
Garlic	S	61.1	22.5	12.4	4.0		
	F	51.7	21.3	20.4	6.6	11.27	*
Olives	S	8.0	8.6	51.0	32.4		
	F	11.3	10.9	42.5	35.3		n.s.
Snacks, etc.							
Sweets	S	3.4	11.1	29.7	55.7		
	F	3.4	9.3	27.1	60.1		n.s.
Chocolate	S	5.5	11.0	25.7	57.8		
	F	4.1	7.2	25.6	63.1		n.s.
Crisps	S	13.7	20.5	36.3	29.5		
	F	2.8	6.8	34.2	56.2	73.83	***
Cigarettes	S	86.8	3.4	5.7	4.0		
	F	85.3	10.1	2.0	2.6	17.93	***

Notes: *** 0.1% level of significance, **1% level of significance, *5% level of signigicance, n.s. not significant.

food item listed, column two gives the nationality of the sample responding. Columns three to six give percentages of each sample responding under that column in the questionnaire. Columns seven and eight give the X^2 and its significance. Similar columns are used in Table 11.3, but only three responses were available.

Food preferences

Table 11.2 shows clearly that for a number of food items there are international differences between these two samples of children from schools only four to five kilometres apart in one Catalan Pyrenean valley.

Wholemeal bread shows a highly significant difference in preferences expressed. This finding would be less important, however, if what is understood by *pan integral* in Spanish Catalonia is not the same as *pain integral* in France. Further work is in progress on this possibility. In Spanish Cerdanya, there is a traditional wholemeal loaf, large and round, which is bought to last for a week on remote farms and eaten hard and dry. Elegant Catalans from Barcelona, on holiday in Cerdanya, have also been seen to choose this bread, per-

Table 11.3 Health views about food expressed by French and Spanish teenagers

Item	Nation	Detrimental	Indifferent	Beneficial	X²	Sig.
Wholemeal bread	S	6.9	48.1	45.0		
	F	8.7	32.2	59.2	15.14	***
Sunflower oil	S	12.9	56.2	30.8		
	F	16.7	53.8	29.5	n.s.	
Olive oil	S	13.9	53.7	32.3		
	F	16.9	45.0	38.1	n.s.	
Margarine	S	20.0	59.2	20.8		
	F	30.6	51.0	18.5	8.43	**
Butter	S	20.2	62.6	17.2		
	F	28.2	41.7	30.1	25.73	***
Milk	S	1.9	16.9	81.2		
	F	2.5	8.8	88.7	8.84	**
Yoghurt	S	2.6	46.2	51.1		
	F	1.9	21.1	77.0	42.98	***
Water	S	0.4	6.8	92.9		
	F	0.6	7.0	92.4	n.s.	
Meats and Fish						
Pork	S	27.6	55.9	16.5		
	F	20.5	51.3	28.1	12.13	**
Lamb	S	8.5	57.5	33.8		
	F	7.7	50.3	42.0	n.s.	
Hamburgers	S	20.0	61.5	18.5		
	F	51.0	33.1	15.9	63.10	***
Liver	S	16.7	52.9	30.4		
	F	13.1	39.6	47.3	17.03	***
Rabbit	S	4.2	60.0	35.8		
	F	1.9	49.4	48.7	11.16	**
Tuna	S	7.7	68.6	23.8	44.7	
	F	2.9	46.8	50.3		***
Cod	S	17.7	53.5	28.8		
	F	14.6	44.9	40.5	8.51	**
Hake	S	7.9	47.6	44.6		
	F	10.9	41.3	47.8	n.s.	
Vegetables and Fruit						
Cabbage	S	7.3	33.0	59.8		
	F	7.0	40.3	52.7	n.s.	
Greens	S	3.8	16.3	79.9		
	F	8.3	18.5	73.2	5.88	*
Spinach	S	7.6	25.8	66.7		
	F	6.0	19.3	74.7	n.s.	
Lettuce	S	1.5	26.8	71.7		
	F	5.1	23.2	71.7	6.08	*
Lentils	S	5.0	46.9	48.1		
	F	4.4	29.4	66.1	19.90	***
Chickpeas	S	8.0	47.0	45.1		
	F	9.5	50.0	40.5	n.s.	

Table 11.3 *Continued*

Item	Nation	Detrimental	Indifferent	Beneficial	X^2	Sig.
Rice	S	2.6	54.5	42.9		
	F	1.6	40.4	58.0	13.48	***
Apples	S	2.7	15.6	81.7		
	F	2.6	17.7	79.7	n.s.	
Oranges	S	3.4	18.2	78.4		
	F	1.3	10.2	88.6	11.39	**
Fruit Juice	S	1.5	10.2	88.3		
	F	4.2	23.6	72.2	22.95	***
Garlic	S	30.0	50.0	20.0		
	F	16.0	44.7	39.3	30.66	***
Olives	S	8.5	70.4	21.2		
	F	7.1	63.2	29.7	n.s.	
Snacks, etc.						
Sweets	S	60.6	29.2	10.2		
	F	76.2	14.9	8.9	18.93	***
Chocolate	S	55.1	35.0	9.9		
	F	50.0	29.6	20.4	12.28	**
Crisps	S	34.8	59.4	5.9		
	F	37.9	49.7	12.4	9.24	**
Cigarettes	S	93.2	5.6	1.1		
	F	95.5	3.2	1.3	n.s.	

Notes: *** 0.1% level of significance, **1% level of significance, *5% level of signigicance, n.s. not significant.

haps in a mood of pride in their 'roots'. Meanwhile, in France, where many small villages still have a bakery and fresh bread each morning is expected, there are wholemeal, granary and all sorts of other varieties of fresh loaves which could correctly be described as *pain integral*. Recognition that these preferences may be expressed about different breads may invalidate the immediate comparison of tastes, but strengthens the overall point of our research into lifestyle differences. Research between groups not only using different languages but having different cultures that can affect such basic items described by the same words in translation, has obvious problems. Similarly, translation advice resulted in the Spanish children being asked to comment on *ganchitos* while the French had been asked about *chips*, both translated in this paper as 'crisps'. Their equivalence lies in their general classification as salted, packeted snacks but despite the advice given, they are not the same thing. So, the highly significant difference in preference expressed should be questioned. It is probably valid to equate these 'junk foods' in the next section where views on health properties are explored.

The value of asking children about preferences in regard to different oils and fats is doubtful, as it is uncertain if they knew which was used. Oils and margarine will not be discussed here, but the finding that more French liked butter fits in with the greater consumption of butter in France than Spain (Vanbelle et al., 1990; Macbeth, 1995). Milk and yoghurt are similarly popular on both sides of the border. Milk consumption in Barcelona has increased greatly in the last thirty years, but informants have suggested that a bowl of milk has long been a traditional breakfast in rural Cerdanya.

Lack of significant international difference in preferences for pork and rabbit and significant differences for lamb, liver and hamburgers are shown. However these summaries hide considerable differences in teenage attitudes to each of these different meats. French teenager attitudes to pork and lamb are very similar to each other and to the Spanish view of pork. It is the Spanish children's enjoyment of lamb that makes the international difference significant for that meat, and in Spain rabbit gets preference scores very similar to those for lamb. *Per capita* consumption of 'ovine meat' was higher in Spain than in France in 1987 (Vanbelle et al., 1990). It will surprise no parents that children on both sides of the border show much greater preference for hamburgers than for liver, but there is an interesting difference in distribution between national samples. Tuna, which we believe was generally assumed by the children to be tinned, is popular. Cod is unpopular. The mixed results for hake should be treated with care. Several children on both sides asked what it was, even though *merluza* (Spanish) and *colin* (French) are far more common than hake is in English. Others may have been content to fill in an answer without great certainty of what fish was involved.

A higher frequency on one side than the other, of course, need not mean that the foodstuff is a children's favourite. This can be most clearly seen from the frequencies for green vegetables where the greater preference by French children for cooked cabbage, spinach and greens is really only a record that fewer noted down that they disliked these vegetables. On the other hand, lettuce is popular among these teenagers on both sides, even though greater preference is shown by the Spanish. While still on the subject of vegetables, it is of considerable interest that French children showed greater preference for the dried pulses, lentils and chickpeas, even though the frequency of actual consumption recorded elsewhere (Macbeth, 1995) was greater in Spain. The suspicion arose that the French children sometimes gave more health-aware answers in their stated preferences, whether through trying to give the right impression or actual taste will not be known. The results for olives, garlic, fruits, sweets (candies) and water are self explanatory.

Concepts of health properties

It should first be recorded that even the youngest of these children had some school education on healthy living, but health beliefs, even those based on a perception of the 'scientific' viewpoint, are influenced by parental cultural beliefs. In fact, the 'science' in specialist journals can be more transitory than the cultural beliefs. Furthermore sophisticated education in nutrition and/or medical science only causes greater problems in how to answer crude health questions such as those found in this questionnaire with its three simple categories. It should be noted that the question, as phrased, concerned 'frequent consumption', but even so, to assign categories of healthy and unhealthy to any foodstuff would be impossible for an 'expert', as the conditions are not given. Three children asked about this, demonstrating their perception of the naïvete of the task. Nevertheless, the point remains that most cultures have traditional views on health properties of different foods and nearly all the children had no difficulty completing the questionnaire. It proved to be interesting that there were so many significant differences in these simple records of the children's concepts of health values.

The statistically significant difference in ideas about wholemeal bread are only made significant by the number of French children who thought it was healthy to eat in quantity but also almost nine percent of the French thought it was unhealthy. One can sympathise with those twenty-seven French children and eighteen Spanish children, who thought it unhealthy, as excessive consumption of any bread might not be recommended. The children have mixed views on the health properties of butter, but this is also true about the medical literature! It is interesting that more French children thought butter healthy than thought margarine healthy. Depending on the margarine, they may have a point, but the advertisers certainly try to recommend many of the margarines on health grounds. No definition of type of margarine was given. The plentiful medical literature currently in praise of olive oil does not seem to have filtered down to the majority of these Cerdan children but as with preferences the children's ability to distinguish any of the oils and fats is questioned.

More Spanish than French children thought pork detrimental to one's health and twenty-eight percent of the French thought it healthy. Meanwhile fifty-one percent of the French thought hamburgers unhealthy causing significant difference between the samples. Generally the teenagers thought liver was indifferent or beneficial to one's health, despite not liking it very much, but more of the French were of the view it was healthy. It would be interesting to know what the basis for the concept that rabbit is healthy is and why more on the French side thought this. There was no significant difference in their views on the health of eating lamb, and in neither country was there a high frequency considering it detrimental, even though the high levels of saturated fat have presumably been discussed in the diet pages of the popular magazines, as they are in Britain. Whereas there had been no significant difference between nations in teenage liking for tuna and dislike of cod, more of the French thought both were healthy. The statistical differences shown for milk and yoghurt lie only in the proportions distinguishing between beneficial and indifferent.

For the vegetables, cabbage, spinach and chickpeas, the numerical differences are not significant. Similarly differences for greens and lettuce are slight. However, more on the French side thought lentils healthy, and had liked them. Rice, which is a common staple in Spain, was considered healthier by the French teenagers. Oranges and fruit juice were considered beneficial by more Spanish, but the difference in perception of apples was not statistically significant. Health values of garlic deserve a comment. In many cultures garlic is thought to have exceptional qualities, and the range is from protection against vampires to aphrodisiac, both of which are presumably 'good for you'. More scientifically based attempts to justify beliefs in the health-giving value of garlic find space in academic journals, especially in regard to blood chemistry and cardiovascular risks (e.g., Fulder, 1989). The French and Spanish children's views differ significantly, but taken together, positive views only slightly exceed negative views and the majority are indifferent.

This small study on health beliefs about a few food items raises intriguing questions about teenagers' views and education, which cannot be resolved on this limited information but indicate a fruitful area for further research into attitudes and information. If the emphasis is on coronary heart disease rather than on malnutrition, then, very generally, it would seem that the French children were better informed. However, to compare these results for some concept of validity assumes that simple health values can be attributed to food items, which is not the case. Nevertheless, in every culture there are pervasive folk traditions about health dangers and remedies, and these are regularly interrelated with foodstuffs. The literature on the purity, danger and classification of what is consumed is now extensive (since Douglas, 1966). For whatever traditional or educational reasons, differences have been shown between these two groups of teenagers.

When collecting the data, the sex of each child was also recorded enabling analysis which showed differences in food preferences between the boys and girls, as discussed elsewhere (Macbeth et al., 1990).

Discussion

Several studies have attempted to build models to show what factors affect food preference. Randall and Sanjur (1981) developed a simple model dividing factors into three categories: characteristics of the individual, characteristics of the food and characteristics of the environment. As not specifically included within 'environment', their model lacks the input of cultural attitudes to individual foodstuffs and is therefore somewhat limiting. Khan (1981), however, developed a model of factors influencing food preferences which incorporates cultural and religious as well as socioeconomic, psychological and extrinsic factors among others, and so presents a more realistic picture.

Familiarity is an aspect often referred to in regard to food preferences, and in fact appears as one of the 'personal factors' in Khan's model. Birch (1988), Pilgrim (1957), Cooper et al. (1971) all studied the effects of familiarity of foodstuffs on the food preferences of children and believe that early exposure is important for forming food preferences. This view is confirmed by Alles-White and Welch (1985) who studied the factors affecting the formation of food preferences in preschool children including familiarity; they concluded that 'food preferences can be enhanced through repeated exposure to the food stimuli and that a critical period may exist in establishing food preferences'. James (1979) suggests that children's food preferences, far from complementing those of the adult population, are actually in opposition to them.

Most research of this kind in the past has looked at the children's subculture as a whole and compared it to that of the adult population. This study, however, did not attempt to compare the food preferences of adults and young children, but instead concentrated on teenagers of two nationalities. While it would seem reasonable to assume that a teenage subculture exists in the Cerdanya valley as elsewhere, these results indicate national differences even between teenagers in one Pyrenean valley and highlighted the fact that the subculture is not internationally homogeneous. There are real differences across this border presumably due to the socialisation experience. Although a national border runs through the Cerdanya valley, this has not prevented movement of people or goods across it. From studies of the supermarkets and shops, all the foodstuffs listed on the questionnaire are available on both sides of the border. This does not mean that all the Spanish and French children were familiar with all the foods mentioned, but where this was not the case (e.g., the words used for hake) the border was not thought to be the reason.

Differences between the frequencies of answers for preference and for health views provide another interesting angle, but ultimately what interests the biologist are the food choices that result in nutrition. Even in 'developed' economies, food preference does not necessarily relate to consumption, especially amongst children who do not have exclusive control over the purchasing and preparation of food in the home or school. One might expect that an increased knowledge about nutrition and health would affect actual consumption, but there have been several studies that found this not to be the case (Axelson et al., 1983; Jalso et al., 1965; Schwartz, 1975 and others), while Shepherd (1990) believes that the relationship is unclear. Furthermore, food selection is based on other factors, such as availability, cost, freshness, hygiene, conspicuous consumption and snobbery, etc.

Correlation of the results given here with those from the seven-day food intake research (Macbeth, 1992; 1995) carried out in conjunction with this study will be discussed elsewhere in an attempt to throw light on the processes that cause differences in non-genetic effects on biology. Our original intention had not been to add to the literature on the aetiology of food preferences, for we had included this comparison of teenagers' attitudes to throw light on the comparison of food intake frequency either side of a border between two nation states, in one valley in Europe's Union. What is important is that differences were not only clearly demonstrated in intake but also in teenagers' expressions of preferences and health beliefs.

Conclusion

These food habit differences have a two-way relationship with nationality. On the one hand they are dependent variables affected by socialisation into the cultures that differ between nation states, and on the other hand food items and specific recipes can be used as expressions of that nationality thereby strengthening the perceptions of national identities. Both affect preferences. Yet, while the processes described as 'culture' may be quite conservative, they are not static, nor are attitudes to nationality or other affiliations. Macbeth and Bertranpetit (1995) have found that recent European relaxation of this international border in the Cerdanya has correlated with a significant decrease, not increase, in transfrontier marriages. It is possible that when Cerdans have no need to rail against an unpopular border, their national differences are more emphasised than their Cerdan unity. Or, one could explain it on the premise that so far supermarkets in the area are still being primarily supplied from Barcelona on the Spanish side, and Montpellier and Perpignan on the French side; that opens up another discussion of whether food retailers and their advertisers determine or reflect local preferences.

References

Alles-White, M.L. and Welch, P. (1985) Factors affecting the formation of food preferences in pre-school children, *Early Child Development and Care*, 21: 265-76

Axelson, M.L., Brinberg, D. and Durand, J.H. (1983), Eating at a fast food restaurant: a social psychological analysis, *Journal of Nutrition Education*, 15: 94-8

Birch, L.L. (1988), Young children's food acceptance patterns, in M.F.Moyal, *Diet and Life: New Technology*, John Libbey Eurotext, Montrouge

Castro, A. (1991) Para un analisis socioantropologico de las practicas de alimentación, *Revista Espanola de Investigaciones Sociologicas*, 53

Chapman, M. (1993) *Social and Biological Aspects of Ethnicity*, Oxford University Press

Chapman, M. and Macbeth, H.M. (1990) *Food For Humanity*, Centre for the Sciences of Food and Nutrition, Oxford

Cooper, J.O., Payne, J.S. and Edwards, C. (1971) Food for thought: an objective approach to changing children's food preferences, *Teaching Exceptional Children*, 3: 73-6

Court, J.M. (1988) Nutrition and adolescents; an overview of concerns in Western society, *Medical Journal of Australia*, 148: 52-6

Dietz, W.H. (1990) You are what you eat – What you eat is what you are, *Journal of Adolescent Health Care*, 11(1): 76-81

Douglas, M. (1966) *Purity and Danger: An Analysis of the Concepts of Pollution and Taboo*, Pantheon, New York

Fulder, S. (1989) Garlic and the prevention of cardiovascular disease, *Cardiology in Practice*, March, 30-5

Galst, J.P. and White, M. (1976) The unhealthy persuader: the reinforcing value of television and children's purchase influencing attempts at the supermarket, *Child Development*, 47(4): 1089-96

Goldberg, M.E., Gorn, G.J. and Gibson, W. (1978) TV messages for snack and breakfast foods: do they influence children's preferences?, *Journal of Consumer Research*, 5(2): 73-81

Jalso, S.B., Burns, M.M. and Rivers, J.M. (1965) Nutritional beliefs and practices, *Journal of the American Dietetic Association*, 47: 263-8

James, A, (1979) Confections, concoctions and conceptions, *Journal of the Anthropological Society of Oxford*, 10(2): 83-95

Jeanneret, O. (1989) Comportements alimentaires des adolescents d'aujourd'hui: aspects epidemiologiqes et psychosociaux, *Sozial und Preventivmedizin*, 43(2): 85-93

Khan, M.A. (1981) Evaluation of food selection patterns and preferences, *CRC Critical Reviews in Food Science and Nutrition*, 15: 129-53

Macbeth, H.M. (1992) Comida, cultural y biologia: comparaciones en un valle catalán, in I. Gonzáles Turmo and P. Romero de Solis, *Antropología de la alimentacion: ensayos sobre la dieta mediterranea*, Fundacion Machado, Andalucia

Macbeth, H.M. (1995) The Cerdanya, a valley divided: biosocial anthropology in a research project, in A.J. Boyce and V. Reynolds (eds.), *Human Populations: Diversity and Adaptation*, Oxford University Press

Macbeth, H.M. and Bertranpetit, J. (1995) Biology, boundaries and borders, *International Journal of Anthropology*, 10:53-62

Macbeth, H.M., Green, A.M. and Castro, A. (1990) Gender differences in adolescent views about food: a study of teenage food preferences in a Pyrenean valley, *Social Biology and Human Affairs*, 55(2): 79-92

Macbeth, H., Salvat, M., Vigo, M. and Bertranpetit, J. (1996) Cerdanya: mountain valley, genetic highway, *Annals of Human Biology*, 23(1): 41-62

Peck, J. (1979) Children's television advertising: an analysis, *Australian Journal of Social Issues*, 14(1): 64-76

Petersen, P.E., Jeffrey, D.B., Bridgwater, C.A. and Dawson, B. (1984) How pronutrition television programming affects children's dietary habits, *Developmental Psychology*, 20(1): 55-63

Pilgrim, F.J. (1957) The components of food acceptance and their measurement, The *American Journal of Clinical Nutrition*, 5: 171-5

Randall, E. and Sanjur, D. (1981) Food preferences: their conceptualization and relationship to consumption, *Ecology of Food and Nutrition*, 11: 151-61

Rosen, J.C. and Silberg, N.T. (1988) Eating attitudes test and eating disorders inventory: norms for adolescent girls and boys, *Journal of Consulting and Clinical Psychology*, 56: 305-306

Rozin, P. (1990) Development in the food domain, *Developmental Psychology*, 26(4): 555-62

Sahlins, P. (1989) *Boundaries: The Making of France and Spain in the Pyrenees*, University of California Press, Berkeley

Schwartz, N.E. (1975) Nutritional knowledge, attitudes and practices of high school graduates, *Journal of the American Dietetic Association*, 66: 28-31

Shepherd, R. (1990) Nutritional and sensory beliefs in food choice, *British Food Journal*, 92(3): 3-8

Story, M. (1990) Study Group Report on the impact of television on adolescent nutritional status, *Journal of Adolescent Health Care*, 11(1): 82-5

Sundberg, J.A. and Endres, J. (1984) Assessing food preferences: a quick procedure, *Early Child Development and Care*, 13: 213-24

Vanbelle, M., de Visscher, G., Focant, M. and Teller, E. (1990) L'évolution
    des habitudes alimentaires dans la C.E.E.: diversité et convergence, a
    publication by *La Semaine Internationale de l'Alimentation, de la Nutrition
    et de l'Agro-industrie*, le CORUM, Montpelier
Walker, C. (1996), Can TV save the planet?, *American Demographer*, 18:
    42-3

12. BREAKING THE RULES
CHANGES IN FOOD ACCEPTABILITY AMONG THE THARU OF NEPAL

Christian McDonaugh

In this chapter I shall describe and provide the outlines of an explanation for a currently unfolding change in food acceptability among the Tharu of Dang, an ethnic group-cum-caste of south-west Nepal. More precisely, I shall be describing events in one village in the Dang valley in south-west Nepal. When I first worked with the Tharu in Dang in 1979 to 1981, buffalo meat was one of the foods not eaten by this group. By 1993, however, the situation had changed to a considerable extent in that some members of the village had begun to eat buffalo meat. When placed in its fuller social context this change is quite striking. I shall first explain what the situation was before in the years leading up to the 1980s and what the significance of a prohibition on buffalo was. Secondly I shall describe the extent of the change in attitudes to buffalo meat, and thirdly I shall explore the reasons for this change against the background context of other related processes of change affecting the Tharu.[1]

In the recent past and still for many Tharu today, and for the older generation in particular, the customary prohibition on buffalo meat formed part of the bundle of cultural markers of the caste status of the Tharu in relation to other castes in the local hierarchy. There has been considerable discussion about the manner in which in south Asia generally diet and rules of commensality are some of

1. Fuller accounts of various aspects of Tharu society and culture can be found in McDonaugh, 1984; Krauskopff, 1989; and Rajaure, 1978, 1981.

the key criteria of caste distinction and, to some extent, status in local hierarchies (see e.g., Dumont, 1980; Marriott, 1959; 1968). In Nepal in the past and still to some extent now, the situation is complex in that foods eaten by some middle-ranking groups were very varied and included buffalo, pork, yak and beef. All of these are in varying degrees low-status foods from the point of view of the high Brahman and Chetri hindu caste groups. This somewhat anomalous situation arises from the history of Nepal, which has been one of a mixing of immigrant Hindu castes with numerous indigenous 'tribal' groups with their own food habits (Sharma, 1978; Höfer, 1979). Simplifying matters a little, in terms of the local hierarchy in Dang, the Tharu occupy a third rank after the Brahmans and Chetris. Below the Tharu rank the lowest and mostly 'untouchable' service castes including the Tailors (Damai), Blacksmiths (Lohār or Kāmi), and Cobblers (Sarki). Diet markers map on to this hierarchy in a way fairly typical of north India and of mainstream Hindu castes in Nepal. Broadly speaking the Brahmans are vegetarian, though lower ranking Brahmans do eat some meats such as pigeon and maybe goat. Chetris eat goat and chicken. Tharu eat all of the above plus pork which in terms of Brahmanic values of purity is a low-ranking impure food. The lowest castes eat buffalo as well as all the above, with only the Sarki eating beef.

For the Tharu, in terms of the local hierarchy, buffalo appeared as one of the cultural markers which distinguished them from the caste groups below them. To this extent, then, they were following the low evaluation of eating buffalo held by the high Hindu castes around them, an evaluation which appears also to be widely reported from parts of India (Harper, 1964; Pocock, 1973). The Tharu are careful to maintain the commensal distinctions between themselves and those below them. So, for instance, they feed visiting service castes such as the Tailors or Blacksmiths either outside or in the outer hall area of their houses and often use disposable leaf plates as well. Any change in food habits in such a milieu would normally be towards emulation of higher castes by, for instance, abandoning some forms of meat and alcohol consumption. This is a frequently reported strategy in much of India among lower castes who adopt a strategy of upward mobility or 'sanskritization' (Srinivas, 1962). Locally, similar reforms were supported by Tharu leaders in the recent past but with little or no effect (McDonaugh, 1989). Their third rank position was not threatened, but at the same time the Tharu lacked any of the other cultural markers such as wearing the sacred thread or hypergamous marriage links with higher castes, which could form the basis for claims to a higher status. Consequently there was no incentive to abandon food practices such as pork and alcohol consumption which anyway are highly valued in terms of internal Tharu cultural values. Nevertheless changes in food practices which would bring them closer to the patterns of the caste groups below them, by for instance eating buffalo, are indeed remarkable against this background of concern for caste values.

So far I have described the Tharu as very much part of the local caste hierarchy, but in many ways they are an exceptional group and stand partly outside or in some sense beside the hierarchy of local castes. Historically, the Tharu have had contacts with surrounding castes but at the same time they have lived very much within their own communities. They possess a number of social and cultural features which distinguish them from local castes and place them nearer the 'tribe' end of classifications which anthropologists and others have used for groups in India and Nepal. It is true that such classifications or typologies are very problematic, not least because of the considerable degree of variation between 'castes' and between 'ethnic groups' or 'tribes' especially in Nepal where there has been a complex mingling of castes with local ethnic groups over the last few centuries (Sharma, 1978). The cultural features which set the Tharu apart from the local castes are too complex to go into in any detail here, but one key indicator is that the Tharu were and to some extent still are seen as *ādivāsi* or aboriginal and as *jangali* or primitive, backward and uneducated by local and especially higher castes. From the Tharu point of view, in so far as one can generalise, they are well able to operate according to the rules of caste interaction, but in many ways they live in two worlds simultaneously: their own in which concerns with status and purity are not stressed, and the caste world in which they have to be conscious of their intermediate position.

Certain further aspects of the recent social, economic and political history of the Tharu need to be explained here. Until the 1960s, when the situation began to change rapidly, the Tharu were very much left to themselves and constituted by far the majority population of the valley. Up to this time the Tharu, even if, strictly speaking, they did not 'own' much of the land, were the sole effective cultivators. Following the eradication of malaria there has been a massive influx of immigrants mainly from the middle hills. One of the results of this has been that the Tharu have experienced considerable upheavals and difficulties, especially over changing tenancy rights and even ownership of their lands. In many cases they have been forced off the land and thousands have migrated to areas to the west and south of the valley. They have experienced economic loss and were forced into new relations of dependency in relation both to

aggressive incoming and also to previous landlords. There have
been legal provisions for protecting their land tenancies but they
have suffered considerable difficulties in securing their rights
through the offices of the expanding local government bureaucracy.
Over the last few decades they have often lacked the Nepali language skills, status and contacts to operate effectively in relation to
the local administration. There are now signs that the situation is stabilising and the Tharu have regained significant ground in protecting
their interests, but their previous and in some cases still current experience has left its mark. In this difficult period of change the Tharu
communities have often appeared withdrawn and isolated, prefer-
ring to turn away from the outside world which has only brought
troubles. They have certainly not been in a position to assert their
own cultural identity, though this is happening now in some
respects. What they could do, however, was to maintain their third-
ranking status among the rapidly growing population of incoming
settlers who have been drawn largely from the Hindu caste groups
from the hills. This outline of recent Tharu history provides further
background to the prohibition on buffalo, but it will also prove
highly relevant when I consider some of the current processes of
change in the village to interpret the changes evident in attitudes to
eating buffalo.

During my first period of fieldwork from 1979 to 1981 it was clear
that buffalo was not eaten, a fact which has also been reported for the
Dang Tharu by Krauskopff (1989: 202) who describes buffalo meat
as 'taboo'. Food was the topic of numerous conversations I had, since
some villagers were curious about my own dietary rules. The fact
that from the start I ate food and drank beer in Tharu houses was
important in helping me to develop relationships in the village. I was
careful to eat everything offered including pork, fish, chicken and
even field rats on occasion. It was known, however, that some Westerners ate beef and I admitted to doing so when in my own country.
I also admitted that I ate buffalo when in Kathmandu where it is
readily available and widely eaten especially by the Newar castes. By
contrast with beef, which was totally out of the question, buffalo was
a source of occasional interest among some of my Tharu friends. It
did not seem to raise quite the same degree of aversion as beef,
though nobody claimed to eat it. Whether anyone ate buffalo privately or when travelling I do not know, but some of the younger
men had apparently sampled buffalo during visits to Kathmandu.

The prohibition or avoidance of buffalo during this time was
clearly shown on the occasion of a major household ritual, 'Barkā
Pujā', which is performed relatively rarely, about every ten to fifteen

years on average for any household.[2] One household did perform this ceremony in 1981. This ritual is marked by certain special features, one of which is that exceptionally a young male buffalo is required as one of the sacrificial offerings to the goddess. Following customary practice in the ritual the buffalo was beheaded and the officiant touched the fresh blood with a finger and very quickly and lightly touched his tongue with the bloodstained finger to signify participation or communion in the sacrifice. All the other sacrificial animals, which included pigs, goats and chickens, were as usual later eaten by the household and numerous guests, but the buffalo carcass was removed in its entirety by a member of a local Cobbler caste household. This is an expensive ritual and the buffalo itself is one of the most costly elements. At the time some Tharu remarked jokingly that it was odd and something of a waste to perform a sacrifice, especially such an expensive one, which they did not subsequently eat themselves.

During a brief visit in 1993 my research focus was not on food habits, but I did nevertheless discover interesting changes in buffalo consumption. In the course of casual conversation the topic of food cropped up and I was told that buffalo meat had now come to be quite widely eaten in the village. This meat, euphemistically known as *thulo kasi* or big goat, was available quite cheaply in the local bazaar town, some two hours walk distant. Apparently Tharu men had begun to eat buffalo on visits to the town and now occasionally brought the meat home for domestic consumption by their families in the village. It was not clear to me how many people did this. As far as I could rapidly ascertain, without going into the matter systematically, this was not done by all households and was disapproved of by members of the older generation, some of whom would not allow such meat to enter their houses. It was apparently a change being brought in by the younger men of the village. Buffalo consumption was, then, known about but still not openly accepted by the whole village. If it was to be done it was still done rather privately and quietly. I think it therefore safe to assume that buffalo was not sufficiently acceptable to be served to guests or provided along with beer to casual visitors during the numerous village festivals over the year. The situation in 1993, then, was one of partial change in the sense that some of the villagers ate buffalo, but it still had not become fully publicly accepted. The old rules still held for formal and public contexts, though everyone knew that in practice the rule was regularly broken in private.

2. See Krauskopff (1989:199-204) for a description of this ceremony.

Illustration of this situation was provided during the performance of a Barkā Pujā ritual by one of the village households which took place by chance while I was visiting in 1993. After the sacrifices had been performed, the carcasses as usual were taken back to the house to be cooked. On this occasion, the Cobblers were only given the head of the buffalo, the rest of the carcass was taken back to the house. The buffalo, however, was cut up and some of it was cooked separately by some young men in an outhouse, though the meat either raw or cooked was divided up into small portions and was given to anyone who wanted some. This meat was not eaten inside the officiating house, where only the meat from the other sacrificial animals was served to guests according to traditional practice. I did not witness the distribution or cooking of the buffalo but learnt about it later that evening, while sitting talking around the kitchen hearth in a friend's house with him, his wife, two sleepy children and a visiting male neighbour. We were still drinking beer as we had been all day since the ceremony, but we had run out of the usual snacks that always accompany beer. The neighbour produced a leafwrapped packet of pieces of fresh raw buffalo meat from his pocket and this was immediately roasted in the embers of the fire and eaten by all of us, men, women and children, on the spot. This was the first and so far the only buffalo meat that I have eaten inside the kitchen of a 'traditional' Tharu house.[3] This whole episode, however, illustrates for me the current position regarding buffalo meat: in public social and ritual contexts it is still not acceptable as food, but in private and domestic contexts it appears now to be widely eaten.

The elements of an explanation for this change in food acceptability that I can offer here must be taken as provisional and indicative, since I have not attempted to research this aspect of Tharu social life in depth. Nevertheless we can identify several aspects of the changing social and cultural context which taken together provide significant insight into why such a change has been occurring.

In the first place, meat *(sikār)* is a highly valued type of food but usually relatively expensive and in short supply. The rapid rise in population in the valley over the last ten to fifteen years at least has resulted in rising demand and rising prices for all meats including goat, mutton, chicken, and pork, the last being the most highly prized by the Tharu. Against this background, it was pointed out to me that buffalo is now increasingly available in the local town and by comparison with other meats, is relatively cheap. Given a funda-

3. In 1985 I had been served buffalo meat along with alcohol in the house of a progressive Tharu local political leader in the local bazaar town.

mental preference for meat, there is then an understandable reason for buying what is relatively good value for money, so long as such meat is culturally acceptable.

Given the predominantly Hindu context, beef is of course completely out of the question for the great majority of groups. Buffalo, however, does not present the same problems at least for the lower castes. There is some evidence that in general, and to a certain extent for the Tharu, buffalo occupies an ambiguous status. Locally, for the high castes buffalo is seen as a low-status food and appears to be associated with the cow. The situation in Nepal as a whole, however, is complicated owing to the ethnic mix. So for example buffalo is eaten by virtually all Newar castes and also by some other middle-ranking groups of roughly equivalent status to the Tharu. This also partly explains its greater local availability to meet demand from immigrants of such groups, as well as from lower castes. In addition, as already noted, Tharu have pointed out to me that they sacrifice buffalo and at least symbolically consume the sacrifice in Barkā Pujā.

Change in attitudes has also been shaped or rather facilitated by a number of processes of change in the region and for the Tharu, especially over the last ten to fifteen years. This is a complex matter and it is not at all easy to specify which aspects of change have been particularly influential. There has been a considerable and rapid influx of population including people from various ethnic and caste groups. There has simultaneously been a great increase in the numbers of people using the new roads and bus networks to travel more and further than ever before. In 1980 the main east/west highway was still under construction through this part of the Terai. Road links to the rest of Nepal and to India were becoming easier but the main highway was still a day's walk from the valley. In 1986, however, the road links from the valley to the east/west highway and thence to the towns of the Terai and Kathmandu were opened so one could reach the capital by bus in one day. People from all communities, including the Tharu, now began to travel to a variety of destinations much more so than before. One consequence has been greater exposure to the outside world, especially towns, with increased opportunities to experiment by, for instance, sampling buffalo meat in distant and anonymous contexts.

The fact remains, however, that eating buffalo can be seen as adopting a low-caste practice and therefore undermining the Tharu position in the local hierarchy. There are nevertheless features of recent Tharu experience which have undermined the force of such concerns and contributed to the confidence to reject or at least challenge such a view.

In the first place, in many everyday and informal contexts there has been a general relaxation in traditional caste-specific food practices, in inter-caste relations and even in commensality. It is difficult to measure the extent of actual change, but it is now common knowledge that some Brahmans have taken to eating a wider variety of meats such as goat and even chicken and some have taken up alcohol. This is true also for local Chetris with whom rules of commensality have loosened so that I have drunk beer and eaten food with local Chetri men in Tharu houses.

Secondly, so far at any rate, it is apparent that those Tharu who now eat buffalo have not become subject to any sanctions or associated loss of status within the Tharu community. This reflects the fact that status distinctions based around or expressed in terms of notions of relative purity have little significance within the Tharu community, and operate within limits that are sufficiently broad to allow for buffalo consumption. In effect this means that those Tharu who now eat buffalo have not thereby been relegated to the status of the local 'untouchable' groups who are the other main consumers of buffalo.

In the third place, and certainly of considerable importance, have been the recent political and economic changes, at least in this village, which have underpinned a new confidence among the Tharu community. In 1980 the majority of Tharu households were sharecropping tenant farmers who were coming to terms with yielding up a greater share of the crop than before, and were engaged in a series of disputes with their non-Tharu landlords over acquiring legally protected official tenancy rights. Most felt insecure and under economic and local political pressure. Over the course of the next decade, however, their persistence paid off: some of the largest Brahman landlords sold up to a larger number of smaller landowners and at the same time most of the Tharu share-croppers gradually managed to obtain legally recognised tenancies. By 1993 the land-holding pattern had changed significantly. Under the land reform legislation, in certain circumstances a tenant has the right, in agreement with the landlord, to take outright ownership of around one quarter of the tenancy land in exchange for revoking protected tenancy rights to cultivate the remaining three quarters of the land. Currently all but a few households have reached such agreements with their landlords. The result is that now most Tharu households own some land, though relatively small amounts, and continue to take in other land on a casual annual basis. The major factor which has promoted such a shift, apart from a strong desire to own land directly, has been the advent of 'Green Revolution' cultivation practices and technology to the village. The introduction of fertilizers, combined with new high-yielding varieties of rice and wheat, and a shift from broadcast sowing to transplanting of rice have resulted in greatly increased yields of rice and wheat. This significant increase in agricultural production has contributed to a growth in economic prosperity, and the resolution of tensions over land has led to a general easing of local intercaste tension and promoted a sense of relative economic security for the time being at least.

Over the last fifteen years developments on the national and local political scene have also contributed significantly to a more confident and outward-looking perspective among the Tharu households. In 1980 the national political system was still based on the 'partyless Panchayat system' in which opposition to the government was stifled. As a result of widespread discontent the king called a national referendum to decide between the Panchayat system and a multiparty democratic system along Indian lines. Locally, the political battle lines between these two camps closely followed the division between the pro-democracy Tharu tenant farmers and the pro-Panchayat high-caste landlords. In the months preceding the referendum, however, a number of young Tharu men, including the chairman of the local Panchayat, were placed in jail on charges relating mainly to the 'safety of the realm'. The Panchayat camp won the referendum nationally and this marked a low point for the Tharu farmers. By 1993, however, major changes had taken place. At the national level the revolution of 1990 had destroyed the discredited Panchayat system, replacing it with the current multiparty democracy. At the local level the most significant effect of this was that for the first time people could openly voice their political opinions and aspirations.

The effects of this change have obviously been profound and are still unfolding, but for the Tharu one consequence appears to be that they have a new sense of optimism and confidence. They are no longer locked into a political structure in which their views and aspirations had always to be kept to themselves, and in which they had for so long occupied a subordinate position to the more powerful and influential high castes around them. These political developments have been fairly recent and it is true that the generally left-wing allegiances of this particular village were not successful in the first round of local elections for the Village Development Committees (VDC) which have replaced the Panchayat as the unit of local government. In fact, in the 1992 elections the Nepal Congress party won a majority in the local VDC. These changes contribute to the new sense confidence in themselves and their culture. It is possible that the trend towards accepting buffalo is partly related to this change in atmosphere. The Tharu now find themselves in a new situation in which the relative dominance of the higher castes is diminished. They can decide for themselves what they will eat, in a context in which caste rules have become somewhat relaxed and the concerns which previously might have pushed them to emulate the culture and practices of the higher castes no longer have the weight and authority they once had.

Ideological challenges to caste and its entailed hierarchical ranking of groups have been more explicitly voiced among a minority of radical Tharu men. Already in 1980, left-wing views challenging caste ideology were expressed in secret by some men. Now such political affiliations have come out more into the open. Opposition to the status ranking aspects of caste is not entirely surprising given the relative emphasis on an egalitarian ethos within Tharu communities. This aspect of Tharu social life cannot be described here in any depth, but although one can identify certain social distinctions based on relative wealth, education, and especially ritual function and knowledge, overall status distinctions such as those based around notions of relative purity play little part within Tharu communities. There are also various customary practices in village communal organisation, for instance, which reflect a broadly egalitarian outlook. This egalitarian view must not be over-emphasised and would have to be qualified in numerous respects, but in combination with left-wing political ideological influences it has led to a minority of men saying that they do not believe in the hierarchical ranking of social groups and they reject treating certain groups as 'untouchable'. They also express the view that differences in dietary practices do not matter and should not form a basis for status distinctions.

Such radical opinions thus far have not had widespread impact on social norms and behaviour but they are clearly related to the new ideas concerning buffalo consumption. They also provide the context for an unprecedented incident I witnessed in a Tharu house in 1993. One evening I was sitting drinking beer in the inner part of a Tharu house with the household head and two other guests, when the family Tailor arrived. At first he was given some beer in the outer hall area of the house which is as far as such 'untouchable' castes ever enter Tharu houses. After a while, however, our Tharu host, one of the village radicals, brought the astonished Tailor into the inner room to sit with the rest of us. Simultaneously, however, the host's wife who was sitting listening to us from the kitchen leapt up and quickly removed all the household deities from the deity room where we were seated. It was clear that she did not approve of inviting the Tailor inside, but her immediate concern was that this would offend the household deities and thus bring misfortune on the household. This incident and the different responses and actions of the two spouses reveals the confrontation of the new egalitarian radical position with the traditional outlook.

To conclude, this short study prompts three observations. Firstly, my material on this change in food habits is clearly limited and in particular this account lacks sufficient attention to the personal perceptions and understandings surrounding buffalo eating held by those Tharu who have adopted this food. Secondly, this case suggests the value of carrying out research over a relatively extended period of time with the same group. 'Taboos' relating to food may not be so fixed as such a term implies and cultural rules and prohibitions, or at least some of them, may be more plastic than they appear in synchronic studies of societies and cultures carried out at a particular time. Thirdly, this case shows that change in food habits is likely to be the result of a complex combination of social influences and processes, and for the Tharu it is not at all easy to isolate the factors which carry most weight in promoting the change described here. What is striking, however, is that the Tharu are living in a period of profound change and one in which some appear able to make choices and adopt innovations which to some extent challenge the values of the higher ranking and economically and politically dominant Hindu castes.

Acknowledgements

I am grateful to the ESRC, the British Academy and the Research Committee of the School of Social Sciences, Oxford Brookes University, for financial support for fieldwork in 1979 to 1981, 1986, and 1993 respectively.

References

Dumont, L. (1980) *Homo Hierarchicus: The Caste System and its Implications,*
    University of Chicago Press

Harper, E. (1964) Ritual pollution as an integrator of caste and religion,
    Journal of Asian Studies, Special Issue Vol. 23

Höfer, A. (1979) *The Caste Hierarchy and the State in Nepal: A Study of the
    Muluki Ain of 1854,* Universitätsverlag Wagner, Innsbruck

Krauskopff, G. (1989) *Maîtres et Possédés: Les Rites et l'Ordre Social chez les
    Tharu (Népal),* Centre National de la Recherche Scientifique, Paris

Marriott, M. (1959) Interactional and attributional theories of caste
    ranking, *Man in India,* XXXIX(2)

Marriott, M. (1968) Caste ranking and food transactions, a matrix analysis,
    in M. Singer and B.S. Cohn (eds.), *Structure and Change in Indian Society,*
    Aldine, Chicago

McDonaugh, C. (1984) The Tharu of Dang: A Study of Social
    Organisation Myth and Ritual in West Nepal, unpublished D.Phil
    Thesis, University of Oxford

McDonaugh, C. (1989) The mythology of the Tharu: aspects of cultural
    identity in Dang, West Nepal, *Kailash,* XV, 3-4

Pocock, D. (1973) *Mind, Body and Wealth: A Study of Belief and Practice in an
    Indian Village,* Basil Blackwell, Oxford

Rajaure, D.P. (1978) An Anthropological Study of the Tharus of Dang-
    Deokhuri, unpublished MA Thesis, Tribhuvan University, Nepal

Rajaure, D.P. (1981) *The Tharu Women of Sukhrwar,* Vol.II pt.3 of *The Status
    of Women in Nepal,* Kathmandu: Centre for Economic Development and
    Administration, Tribhuvan University

Sharma, P.R. (1978) Nepal: Hindu-tribal interface, *Contributions to Nepalese
    Studies,* VI(1)

Srinivas, M.N. (1962) *Caste in Modern India and Other Essays,* Asia
    Publishing House, Bombay

13. CHOICES OF FOOD AND CUISINE IN THE CONCEPT OF SOCIAL SPACE AMONG THE YAO OF THAILAND

Annie Hubert

The theme of this chapter is to show how food preferences closely follow cultural patterns and belief systems, and then to exemplify how sex, age and various representations of space and time structure all these preferences. The fieldwork was carried out among the Yao in the late 1960s and early 1970 in northern Thailand. The Yao's home land was originally south of the Yang Tse river in China. With the Miao, they were the first to suffer the violent oppression of the Han civilisation, which slowly pushed them southwards. Today, they live in the provinces of Guangdong, Guangxi, Hunan and Yunnan. In the nineteenth century, their slow migration south took them to Vietnam, Laos and Thailand. In Thailand, where many groups settled, they are divided into four linguistic groups, and live in small communities scattered in the hills. I shall discuss the Mien, who are established in the mountains of Chiengrai province in northern Thailand.

The Society

All the Yao groups (including the Mien) are divided into twelve original patronymic clans, founded by the mythical ancestor Pi'en Hung, and three others, more recently established. Each clan comprises lineages, which are themselves divided into sections. The elementary unit of this society is the localised lineage, or 'house'. The isolated hamlets or the different groups of houses in a village contain people of the same lineage. The household, which physically regroups the extended family (parents, unmarried children, married sons and their wives and children) into one house, is of great importance as a unit.

The Yao have an elaborate form of ancestor worship, very close to that of the Han Chinese. The household is always associated with a lineage, and with a group of common ancestors, towards whom all the members have ritual obligations, which are taken over by the head of the house, or the 'patriarch'. He represents, in the world of men, all his deceased ancestors. In this society, when women marry they become members of their husband's lineage, and remain in it even as ancestors after their death. The health and prosperity of the household depend above all on the good will of the ancestors. Their help and sympathy are acquired when the living respect rituals during which ancestors are 'fed' and offered money. As discussed below this has repercussions on food choices and cooking.

Based in mountain forests, the Yao practise shifting cultivation (called swidden agriculture): they clear and burn an area of the forest, and on this space (the swidden) they grow rice, corn, vegetables, fruit, and opium. This is done for a period of two to three years, before shifting to another area of the forest, leaving the impoverished soil to regain its fertility over the following few years.

Food and Concepts of Space

For the Yao food choices and cuisine cannot be considered separate from their concepts of space. Their notion of space includes an extratemporal area, or 'nether world'. One cannot consider one world without considering the other; both notions go together and complement each other. The conceptual environment is divided into concentric circles, the centre of which is the house and the village, followed by the intermediate area of the swiddens, followed on the periphery by the forest, and, covering the whole as a vast lid, comes the nether world, or the world of *yin*, inhabited by spirits and ancestors, opposed to the world of *yang*, or the world of the living (see Figure 13.1). This representation of space is essential to understanding the various food consumption patterns. From birth to death the Yao act out their daily lives on both time and space levels, and the nether world is always present. This nether world they see in a very concrete and physical manner and the living are in frequent contact with it every time they address their ancestors whose tablets are placed on the altar situated at the centre of the house. Furthermore, this other world functions like the world of the living: ancestors live in houses, money is spent and banquets are prepared for them by the living. As discussed below, the ancestors have favourite foods and tastes, specific to their 'category' of beings and place in the representation of space.

Figure 13.1 The Yao concept of space can be represented as concentric circles, the centre of which is the heart of 'civilized humanity': the house and village. An intermediate category of space, between 'wild' and 'civilized' is represented by the swiddens. The wild and dangerous space is the forest, while over all this, covering it as a sort of lid, is the netherworld, where ancestors and spirits reside.

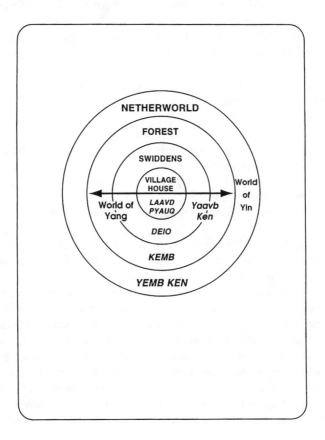

In contrast to the home space, the forest space is considered a wild, exterior area, inhabited by numerous spirits. In the forest, men hunt and people gather wild, edible or medicinal plants. The swiddens, obtained by burning a portion of forest, represent an intermediate space between the wild world and that of the house and village. Practically all the work activities take place there, and all the energies of the household members are devoted to maintaining a profitable balance between nature which gives and men who consume.

The house and the village, the latter particularly, represent the absolute centre of space: domestic, familiar, a refuge for the living. Pigs and chickens, an important part of the diet, are raised in this space category. The interior of the house is divided into three areas around what could be described as the 'ultimate' centre: the ancestors' altar. On the right side of the house is the main room, a more masculine area, the space where guests are received and rituals are carried out. The left part is occupied by the kitchen, territory of the women and children, an informal area where provisions of various foods and produce are piled and where meals are cooked under the protection of 'The Lords of The Kitchen'. Behind the ancestors' altar, snuggled against the rise of the hill, is the most secret and intimate space, where on bamboo platforms, separated by thin partitions, the various couples of the household sleep with their children.

All that is considered consumable by the Yao is covered by three categories:

1. rice, believed to be the basic matter that makes up the body, especially the muscles;
2. meat, which is the energy-giving element, fixed in the body through the presence of rice; and finally
3. vegetables, considered mainly as 'cleansers' of the body.

Alcohol, distilled from rice mash, is considered as the 'spirit' or 'essence' of rice, and it would be a *faux pas*, a somewhat vulgar redundancy, to serve it at the same time as rice.

Raw food is only eaten in the house at the time of a sacrifice. Yet, it is often eaten in the forest (usually by children consuming the berries and plants they gather), and to some extent in meals taken in the swiddens. Non-ritualised, raw food, in the sense that it is not part of a meal offered to the ancestors, has no place inside the house. Things grilled or cooked under the ashes, techniques without receptacles, 'wild' as compared to the civilizing wok or cauldron, are often used in cooking in the swiddens, while cooking in water and/or fat is exclusively done on the wood stoves inside the house. The different ways of cooking and consuming food correspond, then, to particular areas of Yao space. It goes from the most 'civilised' boiled and stewed foods, cooked and eaten inside the house, to grilled and raw foods consumed in the semi-wild area of the swiddens. Raw berries or shoots are eaten in the forest by children, and raw blood by the spirits.

The Various Types of Meals

The Yao eat twice a day, two identical meals: rice and one or two side dishes. However, the type of meal varies with the place in which it is eaten – in the home or in the swidden. Meals in the house are always cooked by the women, and consist of a rice basis, accompanied by one or two side dishes of sautéed or stewed vegetables. One eats on a low table. The rice is served in individual bowls, the side dishes in communal serving bowls and all is eaten with chopsticks. Polite table manners are required. Raw, grilled or ash cooked food are never part of such a meal. For lengthy stays in the swiddens during the important phases of the agricultural cycle, food is prepared in a particular way: the usual combination of boiled and sautéed foods is replaced by food grilled or cooked under ashes. The ingredients used are mainly products of gathering and small-scale hunting, and are served on a banana leaf. Everyone helps themselves directly from this 'plate', eating with their fingers.

As well as the daily pattern of meals there are the banquets and the ancestors' meals. The former are always prepared when a pig is sacrificed to the ancestors. Relatives and neighbours are invited. The men sit around a long line of low tables set next to one another. The meal starts with a formal call and speech to the ancestors. Cups are filled with rice spirit by the son of the head of the house who is always the 'master of drinks'. There are lengthy and numerous exchanges of polite greetings, wishes and other formal short speeches before drinking. The meal is exclusively composed of dishes made with blood and meat, raw and fried. Rice is served at the end, when all have finished drinking.

A major ritual obligation towards one's ancestors and other spirits, is to feed them. They are invited to a banquet each time there is a sacrifice. As food is at the origin and basis of all relationships with the nether world, there is a food offering which requires a preparation different from that for the living. Once the pig has been slaughtered (throat cut) in front of the ancestors' altar, cleaned and presented on a special shelf, the head of the house calls on his ancestors and invites them formally to the feast. He pours rice spirit into small drinking cups and bleeds a chicken, the blood falling into the cups and mixing with the liquor. The essence of the meat (blood) and the essence of the rice (alcohol) are the ancestors' favourite foods. The Yao believe that spirits, and more particularly the ancestor spirits, love alcohol and blood, as they represent the essence of the two most prestigious foods for human beings – rice and meat.

The ancestors are exclusively fed by the men. All of the foods are raw and represent the two main categories: meat and blood which carry energy, and rice (or rice spirit) which fixes this energy. This does not indicate so much a state of 'wildness' or savagery, as a state totally opposite to that of the living, marking the impassable boundaries between the visible and invisible worlds, life and death, translated here by the opposition between the raw and the cooked.

Food Preferences According to Gender and Age

Any discussion of preferences can only be within the contexts of the culture and, in this case, the beliefs and meals outlined above. There are some gender and age differences. Men prepare and eat raw foods (blood and meat) and drink alcohol; they eat before the women and have to set an example of frugality. Their preferences, expressed more particularly during banquets and ceremonies, are for raw meat and blood, heavily spiced with chili pepper and fragrant with mint, basil and dill. They also particularly like grilled bits of meat and offal. These have been stored and preserved in salt in long bamboo tubes and kept for some weeks. This sort of male snack is eaten when friends get together in the evening and talk around an opium pipe and a few small cups of rice whisky. As in many other cultures, men drink more alcohol than women and voice their preferences loudly as a sign of virility.

Women, on the other hand, prepare the daily meals and eat after the men. Their favourite foods are either stewed or boiled. To emphasise the gender difference, a Yao woman should show a slight repulsion to the raw blood and meat eaten by the men. The favourite dish for women is a centrepiece on a table of the wedding banquet: chicken soup with rice noodles. At a wedding, even though there will have been a sacrifice, raw meat and blood are avoided as the presence of these would mean 'blood' between the spouses, fights, feuds and illness. Thus, the women can openly serve what they prefer – soft, boiled, tender and rather bland food. They also love fruit, as do the children. This is eaten as a snack in the afternoon, away from the men. Typical fruits are bananas, papayas, oranges, pomelos. They are a sign of femininity, just as blood is of virility.

After weaning, each child, generally looked after by an elder sister or cousin, will become a member of an autonomous small group, for which the main game and activity consists of finding food to prepare small independent meals throughout the day. Berries, mushrooms, birds, bamboo rats, squirrels, small freshwater crabs, anything will do. Their limited cooking world first comprises entirely of raw food, then of food grilled or cooked under the ashes – in other words the techniques for 'wild foods' (without pots or utensils). Meanwhile, during the family meals in the house, they will also be given soups or well cooked foods.

Children all over the world have a sweet tooth. Yao children are no exception: they love fruit, which they will often share with their mothers and other female relatives in the afternoon, far from the men's activities. Bought sweets are a very rare and extremely special treat for the New Year festivities. Sugar cane is planted almost entirely for their enjoyment. They do, however, also like sour tastes – green berries and young plants gathered in the forest or swiddens. They enjoy ash-baked tubers and grilled titbits, which places them in an intermediate world between that of grown men and women. Boys' and girls' tastes start differentiating as their role in household rituals begins to develop. As adolescents they are supposed to have fully assumed the recognised food 'tastes' of their sex.

Conclusion

As pointed out in Chapter 1, in no society can food preferences be considered completely separate from the cosmology of that society. For the Yao, the well-being and good health of the household depend on the balance and good relations between the interior and the exterior, the living and their ancestors, the swiddens and the work force. Food is at the same time a factor and a condition of this balance, and its abundance is a manifestation of this. It is essential to feed one's ancestors well at the required times in order to obtain from them the favourable conditions for food production. Likewise, it is the type of meal which delimits in time and space, the areas of balance. Each human being develops the proper tastes for the proper foods, corresponding to age, sex and places where meals are eaten. It is part of the general pattern of the universe, as seen by the Yao. These tastes are developed through strong culturally expressed beliefs, and are felt as 'natural'. This sort of harmony is expressed by the Taoist concept of *yin* and *yang*. Health as well as prosperity can be obtained on the condition that this balance is undisturbed. What

outside observers consider to be 'food preferences' can be (and are)
expressed only within the framework of Yao cosmology.

Bibliography

Campbell, M., Pongnoi, N. and Voraphitak, C. (1978) *From the Hands of the
    Hills,* Media Transasia, Hong Kong
Condominas, G. (1980a) Agricultural ecology in the Southeast Asia
    savanna region: the Mnong Gar of Vietnam and their social space, in
    Harris, D.R. (ed.) *Human Ecology in Savanna Environment,* Academic
    Press, London
Condominas, G. (1980b) *L'espace Social: à propos de l'Asie du Sud-Est Paris,*
    Flammarion
Condominas, G. (1980c) La Cuisine: vocabulaire, activités,
    représentations, *Asie du Sud Est et Monde Insulindien,* IX: 3-4
Fortune R. (ed.) (no date) Yao Society: a study of a group of primitives in
    China, *Lignan Science Journal* 19: 341-5
de Garine, I. (1979) Culture et Nutrition, *Communications,* 31: 70-93
Hubert, A. (1974) Cultures sur brûlis en Thailande du Nord, *Journal
    d'Agronomie Tropicale et de Botanique Appliquées,* XXI: 251-5
Hubert, A. (1980) Introduction – la cuisine mien, *Asie du Sud Est et Monde
    Insulindien,* IX: 3-4
Hubert, A. (1985) *L'alimentation dans un village Yao de Thailande du Nord,*
    Editions du CNRS, Paris
Hubert, A. (1990a) Diet, environment and society: cultural and social
    aspects of diet in nutritional anthropology, in G. Ziant (ed.), *Lipids
    and Health,* Elsevier Science Publishers (Biomedical Division) 207-12,
    The Hague
Hubert, A. (1990b) Ethnologie et nutrition: l'alimentation comme pratique
    culturelle chez les Yao de Thailande, in D. Fassin (ed.), *Santé
    Developpement et Société,* Editions Ellispse/AUPELF, Paris
Kandre, P. and Leij Tsan Kuey (1965) Aspects of wealth accumulation,
    ancestor worship and household stability among the Iu Mien Yao,
    *Felicitation Volumes for South East Asian Studies presented to His Highness
    Prince Dhaninivat,* The Siam Society, Bankok
Lebar, F.M., Hickey, G., and Musgrave, J.K. (1964) *Ethnic Groups of
    Mainland Southeast Asia,* Yale University Press, New Haven
Levi-Strauss, C. (1964) *Le Cru et le Cuit,* Plon, Paris
Metailié, G. (1979) Cuisine et santé dans la tradition chinoise,
    Communications, 31: 119-30
Verdier, Y. (1969) Pour une ethnologie culinaire, *L'Homme,* IX: 70-85

14. TASTE AND EMBODIMENT
THE FOOD PREFERENCES OF IRANIANS IN BRITAIN

Lynn Harbottle

Introduction

The word 'taste' applied to food, commonly (especially in nutrition parlance) refers to its organoleptic properties, i.e., the physiological sensations associated with the aromas, and the flavours perceived by the tongue and nasal sensory cells of an individual. Alternatively, 'taste' has connotations (for sociologists and social anthropologists in particular) of fashion and status. Indeed Bourdieu (1984) writes of the means by which the upper classes maintain their distinctiveness from the masses by the selection of specific food items, and James (1997) describes how social tastes and trends in food consumption in contemporary Britain have been necessarily changed and transformed as the élite have sought new ways to reassert their status.

Lalonde (1992) and more recently Csordas (1994), influenced by the work of Merleau-Ponty (1962), emphasise the importance of our experience, not as disembodied minds, nor as a brute fact of nature, but as living bodies. Lalonde contends that it is not so easy to separate the organoleptic and symbolic elements of taste, but argues that even the physiological perceptions of and response to foods are socially conditioned, and that an individual's taste is inextricably linked with that of the group into which s/he is acculturated. Taste is then 'less a matter of *sensation* and more a matter of *perception*' (his emphasis) i.e., the reception, cognition and interpretation of stimuli (1992: 77). Lalonde employs the term 'taste perception' which more accurately connotes the complex combination of physiological and symbolic responses occurring during each food event.

Falk (1994) also recognises the impact of intracultural valuations of foods in determining sensory responses to them. However valid, these theoretical assumptions are based on Western societies and appear to be largely unsubstantiated by empirical data or tempered with evidence from other cultures. This chapter, arising from ethnographic interviews with dispersed groups of Shi'ite Iranians living in central England, sets out to redress that situation. In particular, it follows Lalonde's approach to explore how the food habits and taste preferences, as embodied by this group of migrants, reflect, transform and transcend ethnic, national and global identities.

Migration and Food Habits

Food is central to our sense of individual and group identity. Food beliefs are culturally reproduced (and transformed) from one generation to the next and throughout the life course food is inextricably linked with kinship and with community membership (Lupton, 1996).[1] The categorisation of a substance as edible implies that it is accepted into a particular group of people; commensality based upon the sharing of permitted foods draws people into that community. The ways in which different groups variably categorise foods as edible serve as important markers of difference and have been the subject of great interest for some social scientists (e.g., Bourdieu, 1984; Mennell, 1985; Tremayne, 1993; Caplan, 1997).

For immigrants in a foreign country, some degree of dietary modification might be expected, as familiar foods become unavailable and as dominant food cultures have an impact (Kalka, 1988). Nevertheless, some familiar food habits often remain resistant to change, and maintenance of traditional tastes in food may serve as a cohesive and stabilising force in a potentially alien environment. In the case of Iranians, attempts to analyse the food choices of those in exile must also take note of the heterogeneity of the parent population, in terms of class, ethnicity, and religious and political affiliations (Hoffman, 1990), as well as trends within the host society. In the narratives of these Shi'ite and predominantly middle-class interviewees (and reflected in their

---

1. Although the concept of identity has essentialising tendencies and contemporary analyses focus more on the partial, contingent and fragmentary (adopting the term 'subjectivity'), identity remains an important analytical tool, especially in relation to its socially mediated nature, which is very clearly signified by food and commensality.

dietary tastes) there is apparent a complex interweaving of Eastern and Western, traditional and modern, religious and secular, as well as individual and cultural elements (see also Harbottle, 1996).

Continuity in Food Habits: Tastes and Distastes

Within Iranian cuisine there are key dominant taste themes or 'flavour principles' (Rozin, 1978; Lalonde, 1992) which may be considered to be the principal signifiers or most characteristic elements of that food culture. For example, 'sweet-sour' and 'sweet-savoury' combinations are prevalent throughout the country, as are varied and distinctive combinations of meat with beans/nuts, herbs/spices and fruit. It is noteworthy that the distinctive fruit/meat combinations can be traced back to pre-Islamic times. Hence they may symbolically represent a perpetuity and stability of culinary identity, in opposition to the political upheaval and change which has taken place, especially in recent history (Fragner, 1994).

Amongst Iranian migrants in Britain, considerable continuity is demonstrated with regard to these taste themes. Certain ingredients, such as dried limes, pomegranite juice, *sumac* (an astringent powder) and various herbs, and nuts are essential for this purpose. Although many of these items are available locally, sometimes from Iranian-owned stores, products brought from Iran are preferred. Women (generally the procurers of these products) often justify their choices on grounds of taste 'You can buy them here but they taste funny ...' (Informant A). Although the soils, weather and other growing and storage conditions do have important effects on the organoleptic properties of food, it seems that in this case the physiological response is also influenced by psychological and socio-cultural conditioning (see Harbottle, 1995).

Certain dishes, especially *ghormeh-sabzi* (Harbottle, 1996), which incorporate dominant taste themes and key ingredients, hold particular valence in enabling an individual to *feel* Iranian and to be more powerfully drawn into the group; the different smells, textures and tastes, become 'inescapably embedded in the individual psyche' (Sered, 1988: 133). The link between aesthetics, the emotions and the body's perceived need for food is, in fact, very complex. Although hunger tends to be viewed as a biological drive, and is considered to be separate from appetite, which encompasses responses to psycho-social influences, in practice it is difficult to prove that the experience of hunger is a purely biological one. At times the body may appease other hungers/needs, such as those for love or sex, by using food to fill the void (Falk, 1994); at other times, direct nourishment of the body through adequate nutritional intake does not satisfy the appetite. In this study, for example, some interviewees found that English food did not provide sufficient sustenance. 'When I have Iranian food ... I am not any longer hungry ... it satisfies me, but with English food I am not satisfied ... I'm looking for something else' (Informant B). Other studies also demonstrate how the appearance and palatability of a food may influence the body's digestive response to it (Lalonde, 1992).

'In Iran every city has its own culture [and food] and if you travel you feel the difference from your home' (Informant C). Within the shared (and extensive) vocabulary of national dishes and themes, regional distinctions also continue to be expressed by Iranians in exile (Zubaida, 1994). Differences in taste preferences were employed by interviewees to define ethnic boundaries and to assert superiority over settlers from other provinces. For example, the differences between the cuisine of Azerbyjan and other regions were commonly mentioned. Azeri cooking, especially that of Tabriz, holds an especially high reputation (Zubaida, 1994). Although the region has linguistic affinities with Turkey, the food tastes noticeably Iranian but with its own distinctive features (Fragner, 1994). Azeris are considered to use more lemon juice and butter in cooking than other groups of Iranians, and are reputed to take meticulous care over the preparation and presentation of dishes. Some women (particularly outsiders who married Azeri men) aligned themselves with that ethnic group by adopting their style of cooking and by referring positively to the delicious taste of the food. In contrast, others (some of whom had also intermarried) maintained their own regional affinities, simultaneously considering Azeri cuisine to taste inferior to their food.

Symbolically, an individual's mouth may be regarded as a gateway through which that person guards and protects the self from the outside (Fischler, 1988; Falk, 1994; Lupton, 1996). By extrapolation, the capital city of a country also stands as the entrance point of that nation into the rest of the world. With regard to Teheran, the cosmopolitanism of the Iranian capital city and the openness of its inhabitants to new and varied tastes in regional and international foods (and to new fashions generally) was positively stressed by some ex-residents and contrasted with the unsophisticated and limited culinary repetoire, and the narrow-minded outlook, of those from the provinces. However, in the eyes of some migrants, this openness represents a danger; many Teheranis have been so influenced by foreign cultures and cuisines that they have lost their identity as 'true Iranians'. Hence, a discriminating palate seems to act as a protective mechanism against personal and cultural contamination (see also Harbottle, 1996).

Fischler (1988) considers in more detail the anxiety associated with the act of incorporation; ingestion of poisonous, inedible or taboo substances threatens our integrity at both the biological and symbolic levels. Through psychosocial conditioning we learn to develop aversive behaviour in relation to unknown or suspicious foods and experience powerful emotive and bodily responses, including discomfort, anxiety, nausea and gagging. Data from this study offers further empirical evidence to demonstrate the interweaving of social and biological aversive responses. Although the majority of people interviewed no longer followed Muslim dietary rules, nevertheless their taste perceptions had obviously been moulded by their religious upbringing. Most avoided pork and ham completely (although some would occasionally buy frankfurters or other pork-containing products). Those who had tried pork observed that there was a 'dirtiness' to the taste which they disliked, and most saw no need to integrate it into their well-established culinary repetoire. Few ate only halal meat, although a number did prefer its taste, describing it as 'sweeter' (as well as considering it to be more healthy), whilst non-halal meat was perceived by many to have a slightly tainted flavour.

Even with regard to animals killed according to Muslim regulations, not all meat was considered equally acceptable to the palate. One family described the shoulder cut as more delicious than leg meat, relating this to the fact that the leg retains more blood during ritual slaughter, so is regarded as only 'semi-halal' by orthodox Muslims (Harbottle, 1996). Clearly, the slight ambiguity as to the taxonomic acceptability of leg meat is reflected in the taste perceptions of those consuming it.

Similarly, although some Iranian respondents had gradually acquired a liking for alcoholic beverages, many, not having been socialised into an alcohol-consuming culture, had not developed a taste for this innately unpalatable substance (Rozin et al., 1986). This was at times problematic, particularly for second generation Iranians wanting to socialise with their peer group. For example, one teenager found it difficult to cope with the sustained pressure to consume alcohol exerted by other university students, and the resultant feeling of exclusion if she resisted. Yet, despite her desire to fit in socially, her aversion to alcohol has persisted.

Changing Tastes: Local and Global Influences

Many interviewees have continued to consume Iranian food on a regular basis. Nevertheless, they are obliged to rely predominantly upon English ingredients and it was acknowledged by some informants that the taste of these cooked dishes is different (Harbottle, 1995). Even amongst those who had spent many years in Britain, some continued to perceive the flavour of meals in Iran to be superior to those dishes prepared here. In other cases, informants noted a change in their perceptions of taste, such that one woman found that she no longer liked the flavour of food prepared by her mother, but preferred her own culinary efforts, based on British ingredients (Harbottle, 1995). Significantly, this woman also admitted that she could no longer consider returning to Iran to live and now thinks of England as her permanent home. This illustrates how shifts in ethnic (and other) identities/affinities are reflected through tastes in food.

Global influences upon food preferences, mediated predominantly through travel experiences, the media and education, were apparent in the eating habits of most interviewees. For example, one woman had spent several years in the United States (and had adopted certain aspects of that fast-food culture) before finally settling in Britain. Currently her food preferences are strongly influenced by health concerns (according to the knowledge she has gleaned from studying as a beautician) as well as by an emphasis on convenience foods, unusual amongst the Iranians interviewed. Iranian food retained a residual but important role within her diet, being reserved mainly for special occasions.

The account of another informant (D) illustrates even more clearly the impact of different cultural influences in the evolution of her present multivalent eating habits. In Teheran, her father owned a very successful international restaurant, hence she had become accustomed to developing new tastes in food from an early age. After marrying, she and her husband moved to Italy and they experimented freely with the local cuisine. Her present diet incorporates strong Italian and Iranian themes, and is further expanded by other international recipes gleaned from television. As in the case of other Iranians, her incorporation of British cuisine is limited, in this case to the occasional consumption of fish and chips. Significantly, in the syncretic process, Informant D's response to some Iranian foods has changed. For example, in Iran spaghetti is served in a distinctive manner, i.e., with *tadik* (a special potato or bread crust) and is very popular. However, Informant D now finds that she dislikes this dish and prefers spaghetti cooked in the 'proper' Italian manner.

In this study, Italian food was found to be very popular amongst young people and adults alike and often seemed to provide a useful bridge between British and Iranian cuisines, particularly for mothers obliged to feed their childrens' schoolfriends. The widespread acceptanceof this cuisine, and of Italian culture more generally, also resonates with the attempts by Iranians employed in the fast-food trade to pass as Italians, in order to protect and disguise their own identities which they perceive to be stigmatised following the Islamic revolution (Harbottle, 1997). Perhaps underlying the taste for Italian food is a hunger for greater acceptance and enhancement of Iranian status within the wider society.

Significantly, despite the popularity of Indian food amongst the ethnic majority, it was not highly favoured by most Iranians interviewed. Even those people with Indian or Pakistani friends, and who had eaten in their homes, were not keen on hot food. In some cases marked taste aversions were demonstrated; for example one boy actually vomitted after eating curry.

Capsaicin, the active pungent agent in chillis, is an irritant which causes increased gastric secretion and gut motility; nevertheless, these physiological responses, and the initial innate dislike of the substance, are commonly overcome through social conditioning (Rozin et al., 1986). For Iranians in Britain there may also be, in addition to an absence of conditioning to the substance, a fear of the effects of its incorporation at a symbolic level (Fischler, 1988). The heat of the chilli, the most powerful marker of 'Indian' food, also represents foods of Pakistani and Bangladeshi groups, which are subject to strong negative stereotypes in Britain. The aversion of Iranians to chillis, and therefore to foods from the Indian subcontinent, perhaps represents a reticence to assimilate aspects of these cultures, which might further devalue their own status within British society (Iranians have been strongly stereotyped since the Islamic revolution as raving revolutionaries, Islamic fundamentalists, etc.).

With regard to English food, informants described it as insipid and lacking taste. In contrast, the superiority of Iranian cuisine was stressed, by emphasising its delicious taste as well as its positive and health-giving properties (Harbottle, 1996). In this way taste is clearly used as a metaphor, by which the organoleptic properties of food connote the comparative symbolic value of the two cuisines and cultures. Nevertheless, the impact of local food cultures upon the diets of Iranians in Britain was apparent, particularly in the case of long-term exiles. Most interviewees continued to eat Iranian food regularly, but, especially in the case of those with children, they also considered it important to include some English food in the diet, although there was also a considerable degree of uncertainty as to what constitutes British cuisine. In practice, fish and chips were the most commonly consumed 'British' foods; roast beef was also popular, as was Yorkshire pudding (especially in the Yorkshire region where exposure was greatest). The response to English desserts and cakes was more ambivalent; commonly these did not seem to suit Iranian tastes.

Sweet or Sickly? Cultural Influences in the Preference for Sweet Foods

There appears to be an innate and universal preference for sweet foods amongst humans (Rozin, 1987). It has been suggested that this has an ecological basis – the sweet taste is characteristic of energy sources and is rarely associated with poisons (often identified by a bitter taste). However, '(t)he liking for sweetness, like that of every other sensory characteristic, is for a particular level in a specific, familiar context' (Booth et al., 1987: 146). Although the general preference may be universal, the type of sweet foods consumed shows considerable cross-cultural variation, and evidence from this study also illustrates that the threshold for, and interpretation of, what counts as acceptably sweet is culturally variable.

Iranians usually eat desserts and cakes only on special occasions; some Persian restaurant owners acknowledge that the dessert course is the least appealing element of the meal to British customers. Indeed, there do appear to be major discrepancies between British and Iranian perceptions of sweetness. Iranian people were found to prefer sweet foods with syrupy or sweet-starchy mixtures, often with subtle hints of other flavours, such as cardamom or saffron; to British palates these may be considered sickly sweet. Although it may be expected that the presence of fruit, fat, alcohol and other ingredients may result in a lower perception and greater tolerance of high sugar loads, to Iranian palates 'rich' mixtures, such as Christmas cake are commonly thought (even without the icing) to be too sweet. The very richness which we may perceive as compensating for or counterbalancing the sweetness, seems for them to contribute to sensory overload and distaste (and perhaps underscores the lack of subtlety they commonly associate with British food tastes). However, many of the younger generation (often familiarised through the school meals system) appeared to have developed more anglicised tastes in this regard, and some were partial to English cakes and puddings.

Perhaps it may also be that the sickliness we (especially middle class) British perceive in consuming sugar is a consequence of our own acculturation. Mintz (1985) describes the way sugar consumption and its status as a food have evolved throughout British history, in relation to political-economic influences. Once ascribed medicinal properties, it is currently used in the production of pharmaceuticals but only as a 'filler' or to mask bitter-tasting drugs. In dietary terms it has been demoted from its former, highly esteemed status; now labelled 'empty calories', sugar hovers on the fringes of non-food, or even poison, with its 'pure white and deadly' image.[2]

These contemporary symbolic connotations may explain why, beyond a certain concentration (variable according to individual, gendered and status-related taste thresholds), sugar seems to taste sickly to Europeans – they may harbour deep-rooted anxieties that it will indeed make them sick. In contrast, many Iranians commonly utilise sugar as a medicinal item and its consumption retains positive connotations (Harbottle, 1996), which may partially explain the difference in taste perceptions. It seems to be the richness, perhaps associated with anxiety over the health risks of a high fat intake (Harbottle, 1996) which is perceived as too (i.e., unpleasantly/unhealthily) sweet.

Conclusion

The tendency for dualism, exercised by many scientists and social scientists, which privileges either the biological or the sociocultural aspects of taste, can only ever elicit a partial understanding of the ways in which individuals and groups develop and modify their taste perceptions. A more holistic comprehension of the ways in which these are formed and reshaped requires an integrated approach, such as that offered by phenomenology. There is also a need for more empirical evidence, from diverse cultural contexts, to counterbalance the tendency towards specious and universalistic theorising. In the preceding account I have therefore focused on one particular group, Iranian settlers in Britain, to illustrate some of the specific ways in which the physiological and symbolic aspects of taste are inextricably interwoven in their embodied responses to food.

2. Ironically, fructose ('natural' fruit sugar), maltose (a derivative of raw sugar), molasses, raw cane sugar and honey (the ultimate 'natural' sweet food) are all currently ascribed certain health-giving properties.

References

Booth, D.A., Conner, M.T. and Marie, S. (1987) Sweetness and food
    selection: measurement of sweeteners' effects on acceptance, in J.
    Dobbing, (ed.) *Sweetness*, Springer-Verlag, Berlin
Bourdieu, P. (1984) *Distinction: A Social Critique of the Judgement of Taste*,
    Routledge, London
Caplan, P. (1997) *Food, Identity and Health*, Routledge, London
Csordas, T.J. (1994) *Embodiment and Experience: The Existential Ground of
    Culture and Self.* Cambridge Studies in Medical Anthropology 2,
    Cambridge University Press
Falk, P. (1994) *The Consuming Body*, Sage, London
Fischler, C. (1988) Food, self and identity, *Social Science Information*, 27(2):
    275-92
Fragner, B. (1994) From the Caucasus to the roof of the world: a culinary
    adventure, in S. Zubaida, and R. Tapper, (eds.) *Culinary Cultures of the
    Middle East*, I.B. Tauris, London
Harbottle, L. (1995) *'Palship', Parties and Pilgrimage: Kinship, Community
    formation and Self-Transformation of Iranian Migrants to Britain*, Working
    paper No.9, Sociology and Social Anthropology Working Papers,
    Representations of Places and Identities, Keele University Press
Harbottle, L. (1996) "Bastard" chicken or "*ghormeh-sabsi*": Iranian women
    guarding the health of the migrant family, *Sociological Review Monograph*,
    December
Harbottle, L. (1997) Fast food/spoiled identity: Iranian migrants in the
    British catering trade, in P. Caplan, (ed.) *Food, Identity and Health*,
    Routledge, London
Hoffman, D.M. (1990) Beyond conflict: culture, self and intercultural
    learning among Iranians in the U.S., *International Journal of Intercultural
    Relations*, 14(3): 275-99
James, A. (1997) How British is British food? A view from anthropology, in
    P. Caplan, (ed.) *Food, Identity and Health*, Routledge, London
Kalka, I. (1988) The changing food habits of Gujaratis in Britain, *Journal of
    Human Nutrition and Dietetics*, 1: 329-35
Lalonde, M.P. (1992) Deciphering a meal again, or the anthropology of
    taste, *Social Science Information*, 31(1): 69-86
Lupton, D. (1996) *Food, The Body and the Self*, Sage, London
Mennell, S. (1985) *All Manners of Food: Eating and Taste in England and
    France from the Middle Ages to the Present*, Blackwell, Oxford
Merleau-Ponty, M. (1962) *Phenomenology of Perception*, Routledge and
    Kegan-Paul, London
Mintz, S. (1985) *Sweetness and Power: the Place of Sugar in Modern History*,
    New York: Viking Press
Rozin, P. (1978) The use of characteristic flavourings in human culinary
    practice, in C.M. Apt (ed.) *Flavour: Its Chemical, Behavioural and
    Commercial Aspects*, Westview Press, Boulder, CO

Rozin, P., Pelchat, M.L. and Fallon, A.E. (1986) Psychological factors
    influencing food choice, in C. Ritson, L. Gofton and J. McKenzie (eds.)
    The Food Consumer, Wiley and Sons, London
Rozin, P., (1987) Sweetness, sensuality, sin, safety and socialisation: some
    speculations, in J. Dobbing, (ed.) *Sweetness*, Springer-Verlag, Berlin
Sered, S.S. (1988) Food and holiness: cooking as a sacred act among
    Middle-Eastern Jewish women, *Anthropological Quarterly*, 61(3): 129-39
Tremayne, S. (1993) We Chinese eat a lot: street food as ethnic markers in
    Malaysia, in G. Mars, and V. Mars (eds.), *Food, Culture and History*,
    Vol.1, London Food Seminar
Zubaida, S. (1994) National, communal and global dimensions in Middle
    Eastern food cultures, in S. Zubaida and R. Tapper, (eds.) *Culinary
    Cultures of the Middle East*, I.B. Tauris, London

15. FOOD PREFERENCES AND TASTE IN AN AFRICAN PERSPECTIVE
A WORD OF CAUTION

Igor de Garine

Food preferences and taste can be studied from a number of viewpoints. Neurophysiologists are concerned with trying to demonstrate the role of taste as a mechanism regulating food ingestion and maintaining a qualitative and quantitative balance in the human body through the spontaneous ingestion of substances (foods) appropriate to the maintenance of this equilibrium (Le Magnen, 1951). They are looking into the adaptive role of taste (and food preferences), its contribution to biological fitness through nutrition and, ultimately, to the future of the species (Hladik, 1990; 1993).

As compared to the neurophysiologists, it is obvious that we, as anthropologists can only adopt more modest claims. When considering 'taste', we deal more with flavour: a complex notion encompassing taste and smell (Le Magnen, 1951), and also touch, vision and even hearing if we refer to the 'crunchy' quality of certain foods in some cultures (e.g., Japan).

A further hindrance arises from the impossibility of sharing taste perception. In this respect the observations regarding the United Kingdom made by Harper et al. (1968a, 1968b) on the unattainability of odour characterisation (Harper et al., 1968a) in fact apply to all societies. It is difficult to communicate taste and odour experiences and to a large extent they remain subjective. The social scientist is actually dealing with the verbal expression of sensory perceptions.

The symbolic values, which vary according to culture, social group-
ings and individual diversity, all contribute to the rating of these perceptions. As a matter of fact, physiologists and psychologists also
have to account for personal factors. Physiologists acknowledge
sharp differences in taste perception from one individual to another,
and psychologists have to take into consideration personal life events
when dealing with food preferences and rejections. One is tempted
here to highlight the evocative power of taste and odour in reconsti-
tuting a clear memory from one's past (Proust, 1954). Many physiologists admit the influence of the cultural dimension in the choice of
food (Le Magnen, 1951). Some suggest that taste thresholds may be
characteristic of different traditional groups submitted to distinct
environmental pressures (Hladik, 1990).

Anthropologists are confronted with a very complex field of
investigation and have to allow for the influence of culture on food
and 'taste' preferences. They have to take into account material and
non-material aspects and the objective as well as the symbolic pressures. However, food and taste preferences are acquired within a cultural framework. Children learn to see, feel, hear, touch and taste in
a different fashion according to the society – and the group within
this society – to which they belong (Tornay, 1978). In addition, foods
and dishes are ranked according to specific scales of values through
which each culture exerts its influence.

Sperber (1974: 130) suggests there exists an 'agreement upon insti-
tutionalised cultural representations' in relation to odour. In a wider
sense, we may hypothesise that there is, in each culture (and subculture), some kind of broad consensus about food preferences and
pleasurable tastes. While they may be codified in a cuisine or gastronomy, in most cases they remain implicit.

The anthropologist may have a contribution to make to the problem of universality in the field of taste and food preferences by
unveiling concepts and patterns which are often overlooked because
they are uncommon in our sociocentric Western society.

This chapter will be dealing with food preferences and will touch
upon taste in four traditional Cameroonian societies. Two of them,
the Yassa and the Mvae (a Fang population) are located in the rain-
forest on the southern coast of Cameroon, close to Equatorial Guinea.
The Yassa are traditional marine fishermen who also grow cassava.
The Mvae are traditional agriculturalists with a broad range of cultivated products. They are skilled trappers. Both groups enjoy a well-
balanced diet with a high intake of animal proteins and seldom
undergo a food shortage. For over a century they have been influenced by the urban style of life in Douala and by the Christian mis-

sions. The other two populations, the Massa and the Muzey, are situated in the Sudano-Sahelian savanna, on the banks of the Logone river at the north-eastern tip of Cameroon. They experience seasonal food shortage almost every year and hunger almost every three years. The Western impact is lighter there but the ascendancy exerted by neighbouring Muslim populations has to be taken into account.

In these groups, what are the food preferences and aversions? Which criteria determine their selection and, among these, does taste, or rather flavour, have an influence? What is the relation of these choices to the environmental conditions and to present-day values? Four categories of data are relevant to this discussion:

1. quantitative data on food consumption, nutritional status and time expenditure.
2. questionnaires on food preferences (verbal expression of food preferences);
3. data from direct observation on socio-economic status, daily and ritual food uses;
4. interviews of key informants on the terminology related to foods: taste, odour, texture, desirability, physical and non-physical effects of foods and drinks, and factors involved in food preferences and rejections.

I shall discuss these data in relation to some of the ideas held about non-Western traditional societies and to some of the observations made in the framework of our industrialised world. At this stage I can only offer a few hypotheses.

Among the forest populations we used mostly questionnaires, applied to the volunteer adult males and females belonging to the food consumption and nutritional survey sample in the Yassa village of Ebodié (N=146) and in the Mvae village of Nkoélon (N=114). The following questions were asked:

1. What do you eat/drink most often?
2. What do you prefer to eat/drink? Why?
3. Which are the foods and drinks symbolising wealth that you would offer to a guest?
4. If you had no economic limitations, what would you eat and drink? Why?
5. Which are the foods and drinks of the poor? What do you eat in case of shortage?
6. Which are the foods you don't like eating and why? (distaste)
7. What are your food and drink prohibitions and why? (taboo)

Let us first look at food choices. What are the findings?

Forest Populations

If we compare the data of the quantitative food consumption survey to the food frequency questionnaire, we find that both groups have a clear idea about the use of their main foodstuffs, although they have a tendency to overevaluate the frequency of utilisation of some of them (de Garine, 1993a). Staples and most common sources of protein – for example fish for the Yassa and meat (game) for the Mvae – are quoted most frequently. In both groups, staples are mentioned most often and are the object of positive attitudes (individual preferences and prestige value). They do not figure among negative attitudes. They appear to be offered to a guest, purchased in case of unlimited wealth, and also bought from outside (see Tables 15.1 and 15.2).

Balled cassava pudding and plantain bananas reach the highest positive scores. They may be purchased outside the community and never receive a negative evaluation. The main staple, cassava pudding sticks, also ranks highly but would not be obtained from outside. Alcoholic drinks, especially manufactured ones, are clearly appreciated but spirits also arouse negative reactions among the Mvae (mostly Protestant). Palm wine, which scores moderately positively for its taste, receives a negative evaluation in terms of prestige as it is a symbol of poverty, demonstrating that the consumer cannot afford beer or spirits. Cultivated greens receive a mainly negative score. Cocoyams *(Xanthosoma)* occupy an ambiguous situation. Rice is moderately appreciated; although it appears as a modern and rather prestigious food item, it is not thought to be filling enough. Breadfruit *(Artocarpus)* which grows abundantly, has a very low-ranking image. Green bananas clearly qualify as shortage foods. In both groups, except for the 'wild mangoes' *(Irvingia)* and yams *(Dioscorea)* used in case of shortage, very little mention is made of the plant foods gathered from the forest and which are interpreted as markers of poverty and hunger.

The situation of animal protein foods is more difficult to explain and sharp differences occur between the Yassa and the Mvae. Meat of domesticated animals clearly appears as a prestigious item. Sheep were and are still slaughtered on social occasions such as marriages; beef is of a more modern origin. Fish is frequently eaten in both groups but is regarded negatively by some of the Yassa, for whom it is the daily diet. The situation is symmetrical between the two populations. The Yassa, who are fishermen, have doubts about fish as it is also a shortage food and is never bought from outside the village. To the Yassa, meat appears as a prestige food. The Mvae, who are trappers, would like to obtain more fish, their prestigious food, but meat, their daily fare, is not always appreciated and appears also as a shortage food. It is quite obvious that, although the Yassa and the Mvae are constantly exposed to urban models, they have retained most of the features of their traditional food system. Except for manufactured beverages, the food items they prefer to buy are, to a large extent, their traditional ones. The foods they willingly purchase, except for manufactured beverages and beef (among the Mvae), are produced locally and constitute their daily fare. Cassava sticks and smoked cassava balls are most often consumed, are said to be consumed, are preferred and also benefit from a positive image. They actually constitute the common staple food, what Jelliffe (1967) calls their 'cultural superfood'. It appears that these two groups are satisfied with their traditional diet, which is not always the case among traditional societies confronted with Western models. However, although animal proteins (fish and game) result from predation on the sea and the forest, no benefits are nowadays drawn from the forest plant assets. Gathered foods are no longer valued. The negative attitude displayed towards breadfruit, although it is judged quite palatable, is due to the fact that it is the symbol of laziness and poor agricultural skills. The esteemed staples imply heavy work, while the prized protein food demonstrates initiative and luck (or magical protection).

Let us turn now to the motivations underlying food preferences (see Table 15.3). It is obvious that pleasure and taste are involved. Time budget studies also suggest that the time spent on culinary activities is quite considerable: three hours per day among the Mvae, three-and-a-half among the Yassa. In the latter group the women spend a little more than one-and-a-half hours in processing the cassava pulp into a very smooth paste, which is then wrapped in banana leaves to make what they rightly claim to be the most refined cassava sticks in the area, a cultural marker of their excellency. Both groups enjoy eating and have elaborated a rather varied cuisine, as demonstrated by the number of their 'favourite recipes' (twenty-one among the Yassa, seventeen among the Mvae). If we look into the reasons for food preferences and rejection, personal suitability (as related to individual pleasure) and general considerations about taste come first. However, they are seldom the crude expression of hedonism and usually entail references to health in general and, more often, to personal specifications, for example: '... it is good for me'; '... it suits my body' (and a variety of reasons may be given). Beverages are rated mostly according to their power of intoxication. Traditions and general feeding habits score a little better. Although many food prohibitions exist according to age, sex, or biological state, they do not appear in the answers to the questionnaires. Unexpectedly, reference to cultural change and modernism is seldom acknowledged.

The Yassa and Mvae hold strong xenophobic stereotypes towards each other's food. The Yassa mock the Mvae because they eat leaves from the bush, and are only too happy to consume the rotten fish which has been discarded by the Yassa. The Mvae reciprocate by judging the Yassa's cuisine as absurdly hot, and jeer at them for eating beach crabs, which feed on human faeces.

Savanna Populations

We have not totally processed the questionnaires concerning the data on the Massa and Muzey but general trends already appear. The diet of the Massa is extremely monotonous if we compare it to the cuisine of the forest groups (see Table 15.4). The diet of the Muzey is a little more varied, but there is a lower correlation between the data on food consumption and the self evaluation of food frequency. Early red sorghum *(Sorghum caudatum)* appears as the staple for the traditional Massa. For the Muzey, it is the same species, together with bulrush millet *(Pennisetum sp)*; for the Massa urbanites it is rice together with red sorghum; and for the Fulani trendsetters it is rice and late white pricked sorghum *(Sorghum durrah)*.

Red sorghum, the 'cultural superfood' to which taste expectations are attuned since infancy, is challenged by rice in terms of prestige. Early red sorghum as well as bulrush millet, a main staple among the Muzey, appear among both preferences and dislikes. Although early red sorghum is eaten every day and ritually valued and gastronomically appreciated, it is considered to be the food of backward people. Today it is the symbol of economic retardation. It has also the unfortunate property of producing voluminous faeces (since little of the bran is eliminated from the flour) which look like the thick porridge ingested daily – a constant topic of scorn from the neighbouring groups.

To put it briefly, nowadays the Massa and the Muzey feel less secure, both materially and culturally, about their daily diet than the forest groups mentioned above. The latter have been exposed to modern models for a long time and have progressively found a *modus vivendi* which accounts positively for their traditional food items. The Muzey and especially the Massa are experiencing the disintegration of their traditional way of life and value systems. They have had neither the time nor the material means to integrate old and new ways of life. At present, they prefer white-coloured cereals, the food eaten by Europeans and Muslims. They also refer to ease of preparation in relation to the domestic schedule. Alcoholic drinks are used for their intoxicating properties, as they allow one to 'lose one's shame', to 'be like a lion', and to enable the layman to 'look the local policeman straight in the eye', another illustration of the frustrations they are experiencing.

It clearly appears that palatability and social desirability are divorced. This suggests that food choices and taste preferences have to be evaluated in the total cultural framework of any society.

Looking at the Massa and Muzey has enabled us to enrich the list of food choice criteria which we obtained among the forest populations. This inventory is an open one (see Table 15.5) and unexpected criteria may emerge. Therefore one should not hastily overgeneralise findings, even in the framework of a single society. The same specifications are not required from all kinds of food. As an example, milk, the most prestigious asset of the Massa food system (since it is the product of the society's most valued item – cattle) is never mentioned in the answers to our questionnaire. The informants have focused on what they consider to be the most important points in regard to satisfying nutritional needs. They readily refer to foods which are served at meals in the home, and there may be some correspondence between these and ritual foods.

It also clearly appears that items eaten between meals, at home or outside, such as snacks during specific outdoor tasks or savouries consumed at the market place, are not considered to be nutritive foods. The same applies to drinks. Milk, which is mostly consumed by men during their fattening sessions (de Garine and Koppert, 1990) has a specific function – to fatten the participants and maintain them in high spirits. Rather than being a nutritious food, it is considered as a vehicle for bliss.

All types of foods are not expected to fulfill the same requirements and therefore to provoke the same attitudes (see Table 15.6). There are differences between regular meals taken at home, titbits nibbled between meals, drinks taken on ritual occasions or in a bar, snacks eaten at the market place, foods consumed in the bush or during travel, festive foods and shortage foods (de Garine, 1994; de Garine, 1993b and 1993c).

Furthermore, the same reactions towards the same foods are not expected to be displayed by all categories of individuals in a given society. Children gobble insects, slimy amphibians and cephalopoda, vile foods which no self-respecting adult would consider touching. Girls and women are not expected to indulge in some of the men's foods (which are usually considered too 'strong', as they often come from 'dangerous' animals or are otherwise unbecoming to a 'fair lady'). Among the Muzey, the elderly, who no longer have any success in the domain of love, can indulge in the very strong smelling and bitter tasting foods they relish, e.g., a sauce made from rotting cucumber peel, or the African locust tree condiment 'néré' *(Parkia biglobosa)*. This type of distinction operates also in the forest populations we have studied. Here, the aged, who are not afraid of incurring bad luck in love matters *(awura* in Mvae), can ingest animals which look ugly and wrinkled – reminiscent of old age and impotence, such as the Gabonese viper *(Bitis gabonica)*, the monitor lizard *(Varanus)* or the land turtle *(Kinixys)*. It is easy to imagine why the dashing young males leave the flabby tails of various animals to their elders.

In looking at food preferences, it is therefore necessary to take into account the type of food concerned, its place and time of consumption according to the season and the time of day, as well as attitudes and behaviour in relation to sex, age, biological state (i.e., pregnancy), socio-economic status, ritual situation (i.e., mourning etc.). There is, however, a firm ground on which to tackle cultural regularities in relation to food preferences and palatability. It is the cultural superfood, usually a staple – cassava for the forest groups and early red sorghum for the Muzey and Massa. Among the latter it is the first food to which children are introduced after birth. It represents the bulk of the calories ingested; it is emotionally laden and has much symbolic significance. The various operations relating to its cultivation signal the division of the year's cycle. Red sorghum flour is the basic ingredient of ritual beers and food preparations (as porridge, as a raw mixture of flour and water or mixed together with the blood, etc., of an immolated animal). It is 'good' both materially and symbolically. It is the 'daily bread' and the central reference to the food system including 'taste' appreciation.

It should be noted that the Massa and the Muzey have no general term for 'food'. To eat is expressed by the word *ti.* The general idea of 'being fed' is *ti funa* (literally, to eat the daily sorghum porridge), and also means 'to live'. Nor is there a general term conveying the concept of taste. This idea always carries a hedonistic and moral dimension. *Ti jifia* in Muzey, and *Ti naa* in Massa mean 'it eats good', *jifia* meaning good and beautiful in all senses. *Ti joo* (Massa), *ti yowo* (Muzey) mean 'it eats bad', *joo* denoting bad and ugly in all senses. Terms denoting its palatibility refer to its good smell *(yulumu)* and its taste – it should not be sour *(tlaya)* or bitter *(galaki)* – but mostly to its texture and its filling capacity. This is understandable in societies like the Massa and Muzey that undergo sharp periodic variations in rainfall, which result each year in seasonal food restrictions ranging from hunger *(mayra)* to famine *(baknarda)*. Having enough to eat and feeling satiated is a major concern in daily life as well as in the rituals and the oral literature. The ideal is to be 'full up' *(hobiya)* with nourishing food in order to grow fat *(dorio)* and strong *(vul donota ciw tana* – literally 'gives strength to your meat').

Owing to the bulky texture of the porridge-like staple food, only an appropriate amount of food can be ingested and wastage is avoided. The prepared cereal cake must have the appropriate consistency. It should not be farinaceous *(haskaa)* or gritty *(barsaki)*, too hard *(fu rasiya* – 'porridge hardened') or too heavy *(burdumu)*, nor should it be sticky *(tulbugu)* or too liquid *(nyo* – 'like water'). The Massa, who enjoy a very consistent porridge made from whole flour, mock the Muzey for their too liquid staple from which the bran has been carefully sieved.

Food should not be difficult to swallow *(ti girgidik)* and should be unctuous to the palate *(ti yelwen yelwen)*. Some staples fill this specification and can happily be consumed alone *(los loxio)* or without relish *(losna)* accompanied by a piece of fish or meat. Most of the time the relish must supply the lubricant which allows the mouthfuls of thick porridge to slide down the throat. Glutinous ingredients *(kolboto)*, which are seldom used in Western cuisine, are an essential item in the diet. Okra *(Hibiscus esculentus)*, cooked leaves of red sorrel *(Hibiscus sabdariffa)*, false sesame *(Cerathoteca sesamoïdes)*, and the bark of a particular lime tree *(Grewia mollis)* are used for this purpose. Even though the Massa palate is likely to perceive minute differences in the taste of the porridge, and wild cereals *(Brachiaria sp. Dactyloctenium sp., Setaria sp.)* may be added and that the composition of the relish introduces some variation in the meals, we are nevertheless witnessing a very repetitive diet (see Table 15.4) and a gastronomy which contrasts with the far more adventurous combinations of Western cuisine. Rather than seeking stimulating sensory experiences or demonstrating 'distinction' through exotic choices (Bourdieu 1979: 207), the Massa consumer has internalised his very monotonous diet. He is not as much as the Western gourmet moved by the subtle 'plaisir de la bouche', he is primarily satiating himself. Unlike the cultured table companion, he does not display his wit during the meal. He eats in silence – it is tempting to add as smoothly as breathing. Pleasure, security and well-being arise to a large extent from the repetitive consumption of the same daily fare, rather than boredom leading to rejection, as has been suggested

(Rozin and Rozin, 1981; Rozin et al., this volume). This type of attitude is present in traditional societies even in the modern Western
world, including the present-day rural communities of Europe. In
France, modern Bearnese peasants consume at their morning snack
fried eggs together with cured ham. They acknowledge eating it
every day, claim it is what they prefer as a snack and say they would
continue to consume it even if they had no financial limitations (de
Garine, 1980).

In the savanna populations we have studied, variety is for a large
part brought by animal protein foods. They are sought after. They
are tasty, both salty and fatty. The best pieces are reserved for those
one wishes to honour and for the elderly. Dried fish is most often
consumed. It is 'good' but receives a rather low rating on the hedonistic scale. Fresh fish is appreciated, especially a large fish (e.g., the
Nile perch – *Lates niloticus*). Meat is even more in favour. Domestic
animals are consumed mainly on ritual occasions; their meat is not
to be handled carelessly. Game, which has become a rare commod-
ity, is a rather dangerous item on magico-religious grounds. It has to
be placated for fear of it causing a specific ailment, *tokora*, in the case
of a dangerous animal. Small fish, animals and insects, gathered in
the bush and usually grilled, are not considered serious foods. As a
matter of fact, barbecued meat or fish, which do not satiate, are considered as snack foods. To reach their full status as true foods, they
must be simmered in gravy and be part of the side dish which
accompanies the staple porridge. They should be consumed in a
sheltered household, not outside in the bush, exposed to evil influences. Animal proteins, and especially meat, are less safe than cereal
foods. This is both symbolically, because of the magico-religious
risks they incur, and materially, because they are subject to decay
and often cause gastric troubles in societies where preservation techniques are rudimentary.

Attitudes to Decay and Disgust

The first stage of decaying food is experienced daily by the Massa
who consume each morning the leftovers of the preceding night's
sorghum porridge. It has become *tlaya* (see Table 15.7), sour, the first
stage of decay, and one of the four main tastes distinguished by physiologists. The term *rubuna* applied to milk refers to a pleasant food.
Hebelekna, applied to porridge, and *yakiya*, applied to the previous
night's relish, refer to a still acceptable food. One step further is
bugiwa, 'rotting'. *Kibiwa* is 'not pleasant' but still edible, when drops

begin to fall from meat. At the *cuki jufulu* stage, maggots are present. The food can still be consumed after drying (*soya*) in the sun or in the kitchen. Then comes *bwi* – 'putrid', not edible. Finally, carrion – *tliw mbut ti ngomba* – 'this meat has changed itself into carrion', 'revolting'. This is a dangerous category combining distaste and disgust (Rozin and Fallon, 1987). It is represented in the divination system as *ngomba*, which also means 'death in the bush' or 'unexpected encounter with a dead human body'. Decay (*his bwina* – 'it stinks') is nauseating. *Elele* is disgusting in a general sense and causes vomiting (*vinta*), which is a serious matter involving magico-religious aspects. Any domestic animal vomiting in a compound occasions *yaona*, pollution from an action perpetrated against the normal order, for example breaking an exogamic sexual prohibition, witnessing a ram trying to copulate with a goat. Vomited matter is also used in bewitching activities.

If vomiting is the result of encountering decay, it also occurs through too much freshness: *ngoloma* – 'raw', 'crude', *iria* – 'fresh', 'alive'. Such food is considered nauseating, especially when consumed without salt. This aversion has much to do with odour. The smell for which the Massa and Muzey have a special term, *tledege*, is that of recently slaughtered animal's meat, or of very fresh fish, or the odour of snails. This patterning is original and has no equivalent in Western culture.

Traditional people have to come to terms with decaying foods. The Mvae need somehow to utilise the game they have trapped even if it has remained for some days in the snare before being collected. According to psychologists, the smell of putrefying animal matter, together with faeces, elicits in man the acme of disgust, 'a basic emotion provoking a characteristic facial expression ... a distinctive physiological manifestation (nausea) and a characteristic feeling state (revulsion)' (Rozin and Fallon, 1987: 23). However, it might not be appraised totally in the same way or arouse the same attitude and behaviour in all cultures (Rozin et al., 1993) and in all environments. Dupire (1987), studying the Serer, refers to the overall smell of the villages in which 'unpleasant odours dominate ... faeces, beast carcasses, body smells of humans and domesticated animals' (Dupire, 1987: 7), to which the inhabitants are nevertheless accustomed.

The attitude towards fermented cheese is not the same in the United States as it is in Europe. Northern Europeans frown upon the odour of cooked oil emanating from Spanish kitchens. It is likely that a strong negative sensation would be experiences by Westerners in Chinese villages where human faeces are the main garden manure. Northern Cameroonians, who smell slightly of rancid milk and butter, are disgusted by the odour of steeped cassava so common in the south, and one would be tempted to speak of an 'odour bar' impeding sexual parnership. On the occasion of the ancestors' festival, the Tupuri, a neighbouring tribe of the Massa, consume the crushed leg bones of the cattle which have been slaughtered throughout the preceding year. These bones have reached various levels of putrefaction and constitute a very odoriferous relish indeed. A last example will suffice. Among the mountain societies of Northern Cameroon such as the Fali, the Koma, the Dowayo, the Duupa, the body of a deceased person remains exposed to the mourners for several days, although the temperature is 40° C in the shade. During this period the corpse is progressively wrapped in cotton bands. At the same time, rituals and feasts are performed. The general stench accompanies a period of feasting and dancing which may modify the expected revulsion. The Duupa illustrate in their own fashion tolerance to decaying foods. As ritual gifts to funerals they bring cattle hides which come from animals which have sometimes been slaughtered many days previously and have reached an advanced stage of putrefaction. This does not prevent the assistants from carefully scraping off and eating any morsels of meat which may still be attached to the hides, which are themselves considered to be edible (Eric de Garine: personal communication).

Conclusion

Looking at criteria relating to food preferences among four populations in the rain forest and savanna areas of West Africa shows that, contrary to Western views, groups which have been exposed for the longest time to modern models are not necessarily the most influenced. Where animal protein foods are obtainable in the environment, wild plant resources, although abundant, bring only a small contribution to the diet. It also appears that the study of food preferences and taste from the anthropological viewpoint constitutes a very complex field in which attitudes and behaviour may vary in relation to the nature of the food consumed and according to the time of its consumption and the identity of the consumer. It seems that enculturation plays a noticeable part in food choices and taste preferences and that the major cultural superfood of each society is highly significant in regard to preference.

Finally, satiety and familiarity – rather than gastronomic pleasure and attraction towards novelty – seem to characterise traditional African societies. Unlike that which we notice in societies of overfed

Westerners, it does not lead markedly to boredom and rejection (Rozin and Rozin, 1981). This even applies among hunter/gatherers (see Lee, 1979), to whom a very large range of potential wild foods is readily available. Attitudes towards rotting foods are less negative in traditional African societies than that which is said to be characteristic of man in general. African consumers tolerate and consider edible a broader range of decaying foods, and this is adaptative to their life conditions. Although it may be impossible to challenge the universality of man's physiological equipment and it is commendable to seek common features, culture accounts for notable differences in food choices and taste preferences (Rozin, et al., 1993). A careful analytical approach has still to be carried out on non–Western food systems if we are to avoid hasty generalisations developed from existing data, mostly obtained from sophisticated groups, such as students, belonging to modern urban industrialised societies.

	Observed Frequency		Self-evaluated Frequency		Preferred Foods		Purchased Foods		Foods to be Offered		Food for the Wealthy	
	Yassa	Mvae	Yassa	Mvae	Yassa	Mvae	Yassa	Mvae	Yassa	Mvae	Yassa	Mvae
Cassava pudding sticks	54	47	94	91	56	71	0	0	40	12	0	0
Balled Cassava pudding	21	6	81	21	64	16	57	2	64	0	0	0
Cultivated green vegetables	17	28	0	0	12	33	0	0	0	0	0	0
Plantains	3	9	22	45	45	47	68	15	90	62	69	14
Green bananas	1	6	0	0	0	0	0	0	0	0	0	0
Cocoyams	1	5	0	0	13	28	56	0	12	39	3	0
Bread fruit	3	2	53	11	0	0	0	8	0	0	0	3
Rice	3	4	0	0	24	23	6	13	35	42	5	19
Meat in general (game)	8	35	8	83	13	68	0	0	83	95	0	22
Chicken	1	1	0	0	13	0	0	0	0	0	5	14
Beef	0	0	0	0	0	0	13	48	40	40	0	29
Pork, mutton	0	0	0	0	0	0	2	13	13	46	0	0
Fish in general	74	24	99	67	82	61	0	12	75	41	0	24
Red wine	32	18	20	32	20	36	43	32	87	69	3	38
Beer (manufactured)	48	16	74	56	74	40	100	73	73	27	3	24
Spirits (manufactured)	0	0	0	0	0	0	10	17	47	68	10	24
Soft drinks (manufactured)	4	3	40	42	40	49	28	74	0	0	0	0
Palm wine	14	27	39	39	25	29	5	0	7	12	0	0

Table 15.1 Frequency of consumption of foods, preferences, food items most readily purchased and offered, foods demonstrating wealth among the Yassa and the Mvae. (% of the total number of answers: Yanna N = 146, Mvae N = 114)*

* It should be noted that several answers were made to each question

Table 15.2 Food dislikes and shortage foods among the Yassa and the Mvae (% of the total number of answers: Yassa N = 146, Mvae N = 114)*

	Food dislikes		Foods for the poor and shortage periods	
	Yassa	Mvae	Yassa	Mvae
Sweet cassava	23	12	0	0
Bread fruit	32	19	85	19
Cocoyams	38	32	38	10
Green Bannanas	0	0	40	31
Yams	0	0	0	32
Rice	16	20	0	0
Meat in general	0	37	3	34
Fish in general	37	7	88	32
Palm wine			100	58
Leaves in general (wild)	4	40	8	76

*It should be noted that several answers were made to each question.

Table 15.3 Reasons for food preferences and rejections among the Yassa and the Mvae (% of the total number of answers: Yassa N = 146; Mvae N = 144)

	Preferences		Rejections	
	Yassa	Mvae	Yassa	Mvae
Personal suitability	36	44	39	43
Taste in general	21	11	0	2
Health	22	11	43	37
Fortifying	4	7	2	1
Intoxicating	4	4	10	9
Biological category (gender/age)	1	1	3	3
Tradition	9	11	1	2
Modernism	3	3	0	1
Identity	0	0	0	1
Availability	0	0	0	1

Table 15.4 Frequency of dishes consumed at meals among the
Massa (*Source:* Koppert 1981).

	Frequency	%
Thick sorghum or millet porridge	861	42.3
Relish, mostly with dried fish and okra	740	36.3
Barbecued fish	155	7.6
Milk	140	6.9
Sorghum or millet gruel	73	3.6
Meat	17	0.8
Tubers	7	0.3
Other dishes	44	2.2
Total	2,036	100%

Table 15.5 Criteria for food choices in increasing order of frequency (*mentioned to *****mentioned very often)

"Flavour"	Odour (in general)**
	Degree of freshness**
	Texture***
	Taste****
	Individual suitability*****
	Colour**
	Physical temperature**
	Hot/cold symbolic division**
Health	Association with disease**
Nutrition	Digestive properties***
	Strengthening***
	Satiating****
	Fattening****
Affect related to:	Happiness/unhappiness*
	Abundance/hunger*
Psychological properties	Courage/cowardice*
	Loss of shame*
Economic adequacy	Availability*
	Affluence*
	Price*
Cultural adequacy	Traditional*
	Foreign, modern*
Social adequacy	Kinship*
	Socio-economic status*
	Religion*
Biological adequacy	Age*
	Sex*
	Biological status*
Magico-religious adequacy in relation to:	Ritual episodes*
	Taboos*
	Physical disease*
	Magical stress*

Table 15.6 Other aspects to be considered in food evaluation

Type of food   Staple
                                                    Relish
                                                    Snack foods
                                                    Children's foods
                                                    "Hunger" foods
                                                    Famine foods
                                                    Alcoholic drinks
                                                    Soft drinks
                                                    Drink

Place of consumption   Home
                                                    Village
                                                    Market
                                                    Foreign place

Time of consumption in reference to: The day
                                                    The season

Local word	Tledege	Ngoloma	Tlaya	Bugiya	Cuki jufulu	Soo	Bwi	Hahana	Mbut ti ngomba
Description of substance	Too raw	Fresh	Sour *Rubuna* (sour milk) *Hebelekna* (sour porridge) *Yakiya* (sour relish)	Beginning to rot	Maggots appear	Dried after beginning to rot	Rotten	Putrid	Changed into carrion
Description of reaction	Nauseating	Appetizing	Edible	Hardly edible	Not edible without drying	Acceptable	Barely edible	Inedible	Nauseating
scale (– negative and + positive)	–	++	+	–	– –	–	– –	– – –	– – – –

Table 15.7 Evaluation of stages of decay and of disgust among the Massa and Muzey in increasing order from left to right

References

Bourdieu, P. (1979) *La Distinction: Critique Sociale du Jugement*, Editions de Minuit, Paris

de Garine, I. (1980) Une anthropologie alimentaire des Français, *Ethnologie Française*, N.S. 10(3): 227-38

de Garine, I. (1993a) Food resources and preferences in the Cameroonian Forest, in C.M. Hladik, H. Pagezy, O.F. Linares, A. Hladik, A. Semple and M. Hadley (eds.), *Food and Nutrition in the Tropical Forest. Proceedings of Unesco Symposium on Food and Nutrition in the Tropical Forest: Biocultural Interactions and Applications to Development*, Man and the Biosphere Series, Unesco, Paris, 15: 561-75

de Garine, I. (1993b) Contribution of wild food resources to the solution of food crises, in H-G. Bohle, T.E. Downing, J.O. Field and F.N. Ibrahim (eds.), *Coping with Vulnerability and Criticality: Case Studies on Food-Insecure Groups and Regions*, Breitenbach verlag, Saarbrücken, 339-59

de Garine, I. (1993c) Coping strategies in case of hunger of the most vulnerable groups among the Massa and Mussey of Northern Cameroon, *Geo Journal*, Kluwer Academic Publishers, London, 30(2): 159-66

de Garine, I. (1994) The diet and nutrition of human populations, in T. Ingold (ed.), *Humanity, Culture and Social Life: An Encyclopaedia of Anthropology*, Routledge Publishers, London, 226-66

de Garine, I. and Koppert, G.J.A. (1990) Social adaptation to season and uncertainty in food supply, in G.A. Harrison and J.C. Waterlow (eds.), *Diet and Disease in Traditional and Developing Societies*, Cambridge University Press, 240-89

Dupire, M. (1987) Des goûts et des odeurs: classification et universaux, *L'Homme*, 27(104): 5-26

Harper, R., Land, D.G., Griffith, N.M. and Bate-Smith, E.C., (1968a) Odour qualities: a glossary of usage, *British Journal of Psychology*, 59(3): 231-52

Harper, R., Bate-Smith, E.C., Land, D.G. and Griffith, N.M. (1968b) *A glossary of odour stimuli and their qualities, Perfumery and Essential Oil Record*, London, January, 1-16

Hladik, C.M., (1990) Gustatory perception and food taste, in C.M. Hladik, S. Bahuchet and I. de Garine (eds.), *Food and Nutrition in the African Rain Forest*, CNRS, Unesco/Mab., Paris

Hladik, C.M. (1993) Fruits of the rain forest and gustatory perception as a result of evolutionary interactions, in C.M. Hladik, H. Pagezy, O.F. Linares, A. Hladik, A. Semple and M. Hadley (eds.), *Food and Nutrition in the Tropical Forest*, Proceedings of UNESCO Symposium on Food and Nutrition in the Tropical Forest: Biocultural Interactions and Applications to Development, Man and the Biosphere Series, UNESCO, Paris, 15: 9

Jelliffe, D.B. (1967) Parallel food classifications in developing and industrialised countries, *American Journal of Nutrition*, 2(3): 273-81

Koppert, G. (1981) *Kogoyna, Etude Alimentaire, Anthropométrique et Pathologique d'un Village Massa du Nord Cameroun*, Département de Nutrition, Université des Sciences Agronomiques, Wageningen, Pays Bas, Miméo

Lee, R.B. (1979) *The !Kung San: Men, Women and Work in a Foraging Society*, Cambridge University Press

Le Magnen, J. (1951) *Le Goût et les Saveurs*, Presses Universitaires de France, Paris

Proust, M., (1954) *A la Recherche du Temps Perdu*, Gallimard, Paris

Rozin, E. and Rozin, P. (1981) Culinary themes and variations, *Natural History*, American Museum of Natural History, 90(2): 6-14

Rozin, P. and Fallon, A.E. (1987) A perspective on disgust, *Psychological Review*, 94(1): 23-41

Rozin, P., Haidt, J. and McCauley, C.R. (1993) Disgust, in M. Lewis and J. Haviland (eds.) *Handbook of Emotions*, Guildford, New York, 575-94

Sperber, D. (1974) *Le Symbolisme en Général*, Herman, Paris

Tornay, S. (1978) (ed.) *Voir et Nommer les Couleurs: Introduction*, Laboratoire d'Ethnologie et de Sociologie Comparative, Université de Paris X, Nanterre, IX-LI

NOTES ON CONTRIBUTORS

Igor de Garine is Director of Research at CNRS (National Centre for Scientific Research, France), and responsible for the research group UMR 9935 Anthropology and Ethnology of Food. He is also President of the International Commission on the Anthropology of Food (ICAF) within the framework of the International Union for Anthropological and Ethnological Sciences (IUAES).

Isabel Gonzalez Turmo is Associate Professor in the Department of Social Anthropology at the University of Seville. She has specialised in the anthropology of food and nutrition, and on the anthropology of fishing, having worked on Andalucian and Mediterranean perspectives. She has published several books.

Alex Green is a graduate of Oxford Brookes University, Oxford, who worked as research assistant to Helen Macbeth on the study of food habits in the Cerdanya valley.

Jonathan Haidt is Assistant Professor of Psychology at the University of Virginia, Charlottesville, Virginia. His field of interest is the cultural psychology of the emotions.

Lynn Harbottle is a medical anthropologist and nutritionist. She has worked in Papua New Guinea and with the U.K. National Health Service. Her research includes a dietary survey of British Pakistani and Bangladeshi weanlings, and work among Iranian settlers in Britain concerning the use of food as a marker of identity. She lectures at the University of Keele, Department of Sociology and Social Anthropology.

Claude Marcel Hladik, with Bruno Simmen, works on feeding behaviour in an interdisciplinary research team 'Anthropologie et Ecologie de l'Alimentation' at the Muséum National d'Histoire Naturelle (Brunoy, France). Before creating this CNRS research unit in cooperation with anthropologists, he carried out fieldwork to characterize dietary adaptations and feeding behaviour of wild primates in Africa, America and Asia.

Annie Hubert is a Research Director of the CNRS (National Centre for Scientific Research, France), currently working in the Laboratoire de Santé, Société et Développement, at the University of Bordeaux. She has specialised in nutritional anthropology and the anthropology of health, and has carried out research in Thailand, Morocco and France.

Rebecca Huss-Ashmore is a nutritional and medical anthropologist interested in human adaptability and human population biology. She has worked on changing patterns of food consumption in eastern and southern Africa. Her current interests include coping strategies of people in peri-urban environments in the U.S. and Africa, and the role of environmental perception in effective human adaptation to new environments.

Sumio Imada is Associate Professor of Psychology at Hiroshima Shudo University, Hiroshima. He is a psychologist interested in food.

Susan Johnston is a medical anthropologist and human biologist. She is interested in questions of dietary change and traditional use of wild plants as food and medicine. Her current research involves looking at changing diet, lifestyle, and chronic disease patterns for a Native American population, the Blackfeet of Montana.

Sue Lawry is a graduate of Oxford Brookes University, Oxford, who worked as assistant to Helen Macbeth in regard to the *Food Preferences and Taste* conference and this volume.

Helen Macbeth is Principal Lecturer in Anthropology, Oxford Brookes University, Oxford. She is Chair of ICAF (Europe) and of the Biosocial Society. Both in teaching and research she has worked to bring perspectives from biological and social anthropology together. She is Editor of the journal, *Social Biology and Human Affairs*.

Clark McCauley is Professor of Psychology at Bryn Mawr College, Bryn Mawr, Pennsylvania. His field is social psychology.

Christian McDonaugh is a Senior Lecturer in Social Anthropology at Oxford Brookes University. His main interests include the ethnography of ethnic groups in Nepal, and the application of anthropology in policy and practice.

Ellen Messer is an anthropologist and past Director in the World Hunger Program at Brown University, Providence, Rhode Island. Her publications include *Anthropological Perspectives on Diet* (1984) and *Anthropology and Human Rights, Annual Review of Anthropology* (1993). She is co-author and co-editor of the biannual *Hunger Report* issued by the World Hunger Program.

Edmund Rolls is Professor of Experimental Psychology at the University of Oxford, Department of Experimental Psychology. He is Associate Director of the Medical Research Council Oxford Interdisciplinary Research Centre for Cognitive Neuroscience, and a Fellow of Corpus Christi College. His research interests include the neurophysiology of vision, the neurophysiology of taste, olfaction and feeding, neural mechanisms of memory and emotion, the neurophysiology of the striatum and the operation of real neuronal networks in the brain.

Paul Rozin is the Edmund J. and Julia W Kahn Professor in Psychology at the University of Pennsylvania. He has served as editor of the journal *Appetite*, and has been the recipient of a Guggenheim Fellowship, and two fellowship appointments at the Center for Advanced Study in Behavioral Sciences at Stanford. His research focuses on biological, psychological and cultural determinants of human food choice, with particular emphases on disgust and contagion, the acquisition of likes for foods, and cultural differences in the way food functions in life.

Wulf Schiefenhövel, M.D. is Professor at the University of Munich, and research associate with the Research Group for Human Ethology in the Max Planck Institute, Andechs. He has carried out long-term field research in Papua New Guinea and Irian Jaya on topics which include ethnomedicine, birth behaviour, infancy, non-verbal communication, chronobiology and Austronesian migrations.

Bruno Simmen, with Claude Marcel Hladik, works on feeding behaviour in an interdisciplinary research team 'Anthropologie et Ecologie de l'Alimentation' at the Muséum National d'Histoire Naturelle (Brunoy, France). His research focuses on primate taste perception, combining observation of wild primates, mostly in French Guiana, and behavioural experiments at the Brunoy laboratory.

Manuela Valagao is Lecturer in the Sociology of Food and Environment at the ISCTE (Higher Institute of the Sciences of Labour and Business), University of Lisbon. She is a researcher with INIA (National Institute for Agricultural Research, Portugal) on questions of food change in rural environments.

INDEX